Rachel Ama's Vegan Eats

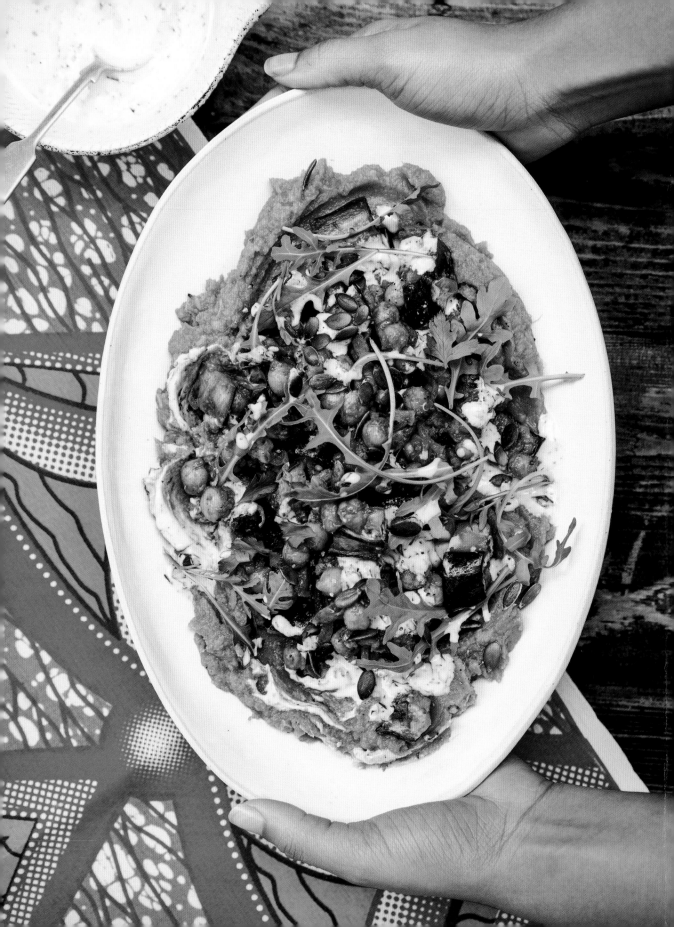

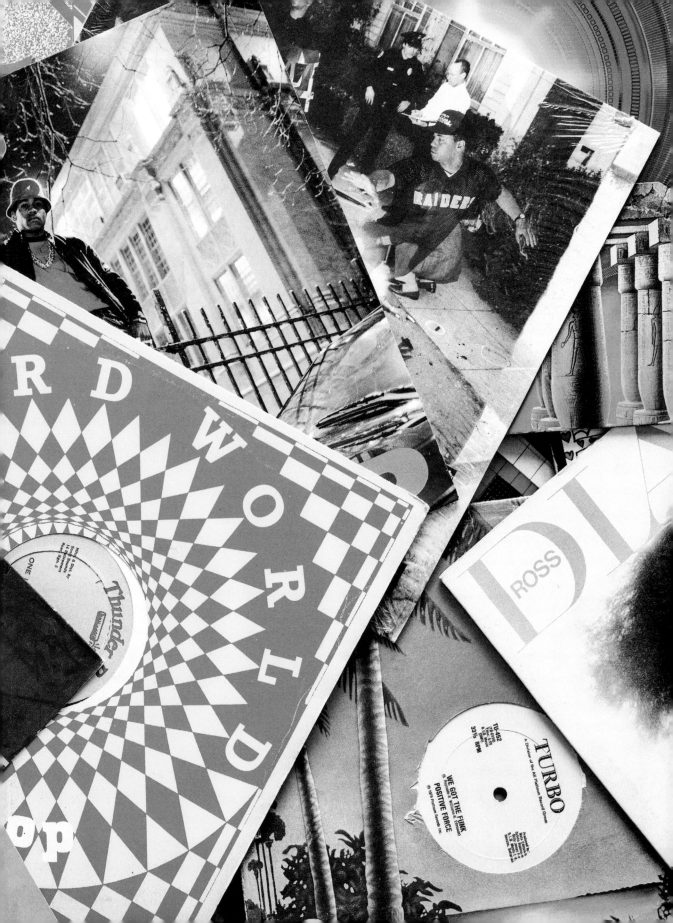

RACHEL AMA'S VEGAN EATS

TASTY PLANT-BASED RECIPES FOR EVERY DAY

EBURY PRESS

Contents

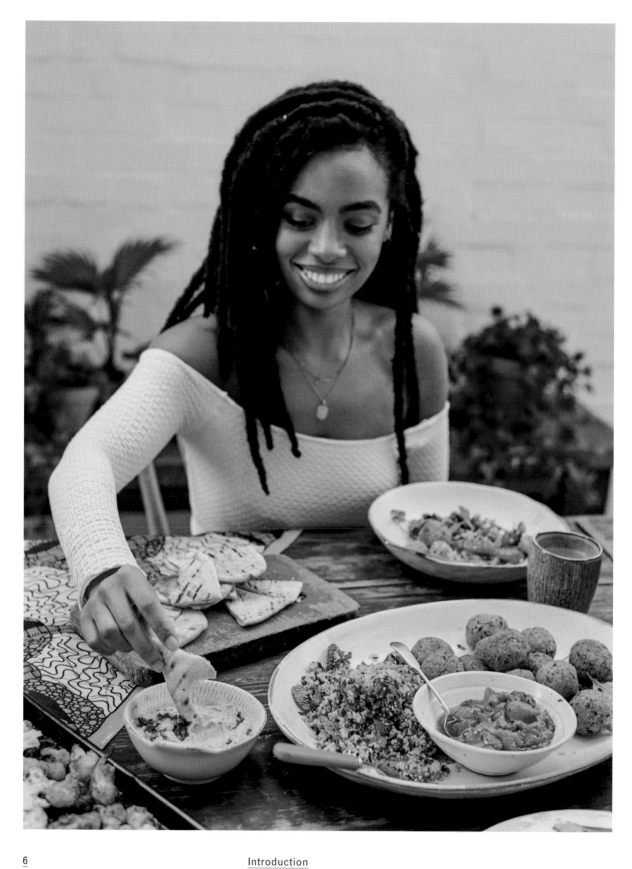

Introduction

Introduction

Thank you for buying my first book! I can't believe it's finally out there, and that it is full of all of my favourite flavours and recipes. In fact it's full of all of my favourite things – which (as some of you may already know) are mainly either connected to food or music.

Since my journey into cooking and eating vegan food began, I have been on a mission to create recipes that are full of flavour, texture, spice and comfort. That's the way I like to cook – the way I was brought up to eat and enjoy food – and I didn't want that to change just because I was no longer eating animal products.

So how did this all begin for me? I grew up in a relatively health-conscious household and although I still opted for trips to KFC and chicken shops after school, things like fizzy drinks, sweets and processed foods were not a frequent feature in my house. Luckily for me, although my mum was running her business as we were growing up she still made time to cook us meals from scratch (thank you Mum!), with maybe a take-out on a Friday here and there – she'd call it her break from the kitchen. Around 10 or so years ago my mum got even more into nutrition and went on to study it, which meant that the variety of fresh fruits and vegetables and seeds in my house was increasing by the day. I used to call her juices her potions because they were always made with things I'd never heard of, especially her green, sometimes brown, ones. And then there were all these different powders which she added to her food, such as moringa and baobab, for added vitamins and nutrients. But we still ate meat, fish and dairy.

As a teenager I started struggling with digestive problems and really intense stomach pains to the point where I'd be out with friends and have to go home when I'd just cry from the pain. But it wasn't until I went to university where I went on a dairy overload – think pasta coated in cheese, lots of cheese, and pizzas dripping in cheese – that I started to get really unwell. My digestion was awful and with that I had a list of painful problems that doctors and multiple specialists couldn't figure out. Luckily Mum, my holistic health guru, suggested that I was lactose intolerant. I was really hoping she was wrong and it wasn't dairy causing the problems, as 10 years ago all the dairy-free alternatives weren't around and I loved hot chocolate and cheese! However, I was in so much pain and agony that I knew I'd do anything to figure out the cause. So I completely cut out dairy from my diet and within a few months my body really started to heal – it was genuinely amazing.

A few years later I found myself curious about vegan diets as I'd heard about them briefly in conversations here and there. The conversations were usually like,

'You heard of the vegan thing?'

'Yeah, I don't really get it, chicken is great.'

'Yeah, me either...'

And that's as far as the general group chats would go, but I was still slightly intrigued as I didn't know any vegans or really understand why people went vegan.

Not long after, I was talking to someone about my vegan curiosity and how we both didn't quite understand it as a lifestyle choice. They'd seen some documentaries and suggested them to me, and thanks to Netflix, I went on a documentary spiral looking at animal farming and I was immediately heartbroken. I've always considered myself an animal lover, having had pets all of my life, but I'd never made the association between my pets, animals and the food I ate. I'd always been taught and believed that meat, fish and dairy were human fuel and that it was normal and natural to eat them. But after watching multiple documentaries my perspective changed. I'd finally seen what really happens in factories and how my KFC chicken wings after school had ended up on my plate, and I was completely devastated. The next day I went vegan.

I often get asked if I found the switch hard, and honestly, it felt natural and normal for me, but I know it doesn't feel that way for everyone. I'd already been surrounded by so many different nutrient-rich foods (thanks Mum), and I'd already stopped eating dairy, so all I needed to cut out was fish and meat.

The thing I did struggle with at the beginning was eating enough food; I found myself hungry at night, which was really annoying. A hangry Rachel isn't that fun to be around. I was eating so many vegetables but I wasn't getting enough calories. I soon realised that I needed to add more filling foods with a variety of legumes, grains, nuts and seeds into my meals to fuel my body properly. Once I'd done this – problem solved!

My initial go-tos were vegan pesto pasta with cherry tomatoes, or hummus and pitta. I already loved these meals, plus they're versatile as you can keep them basic or make them fancy by adding more vegetables and nuts. I love hummus in a pitta with grilled vegetables and fresh salad sandwiches – yum – but I was excited to see what other meals I could create. So what really changed for me when I became vegan was this new passion and enthusiasm I developed around cooking. I asked myself how I could continue to make piff (peng/banging/delicious) food but without the meat and fish and dairy and it became my mission.

As well as having African, Welsh and Caribbean roots, growing up in London I was surrounded by different cultures and cuisines. When I went vegan, I wanted to continue to eat all the flavours and meals that I used to love, so I started experimenting with the same seasonings and spices but using plant-based food. I also looked at how I could cook vegetables in different ways to bring out a variety of textures. My favourite way to create meals is to use whole, plant-based foods with as many colours as possible – the more colour the greater the variety of nutrients, textures and flavours. Also, a beige plate was never my kind of plate.

When I first went vegan I would look on YouTube for inspiration but I didn't find anyone I could relate to, or who cooked the foods I was used to eating. I really wanted to share how much I was loving my vegan food with my friends and family – and convince them it was more than just kale and celery, which is what they thought! – so that is why I started sharing recipes publicly. I really do believe that plant-based eating is good for the animals, our health and the environment. So I decided that my own little branch of activism would be to share recipes on YouTube to help or inspire anyone thinking about plant-based eating who wasn't sure what food to make. I also hoped to give long-term vegans some more ideas. Now, with this book, I get to share over 100 vegan recipes with you!

The book really translates my flavour palate through a range of plant-based recipes. There are everyday essential classics such as lasagne, curries and stews that are quick and easy to make for your weekday meals. You'll find staple lunches like a jacket potato and 'chuna', which is great for your friends that miss their tuna – trust me, my version tastes amazing – and really flavoursome sandwiches, salads and wraps that can also be prepped in advance for lunch the next day. I've also put in some really delicious recipes that take inspiration from typical meat dishes but are made with vegetables instead. Things like my Spiced Griddled Aubergine Kebabs (see page 102) – it takes a little longer to make but is a definite showstopper and well worth it! And, one of my favourites: the Crispy Jerk Barbecue Tacos (see page 127) with sweet plantain and fresh slaw for all the Caribbean feels. I love the way Caribbean flavours and spices make my kitchen smell; they remind me of my grandma's house and she was an incredible cook. I wish I could share the kitchen with her now.

I have put together a little store cupboard glossary at the back of the book, which has some useful ingredients for vegan cooking and also explains some of the ingredients I use in my recipes in case you want to know a little bit

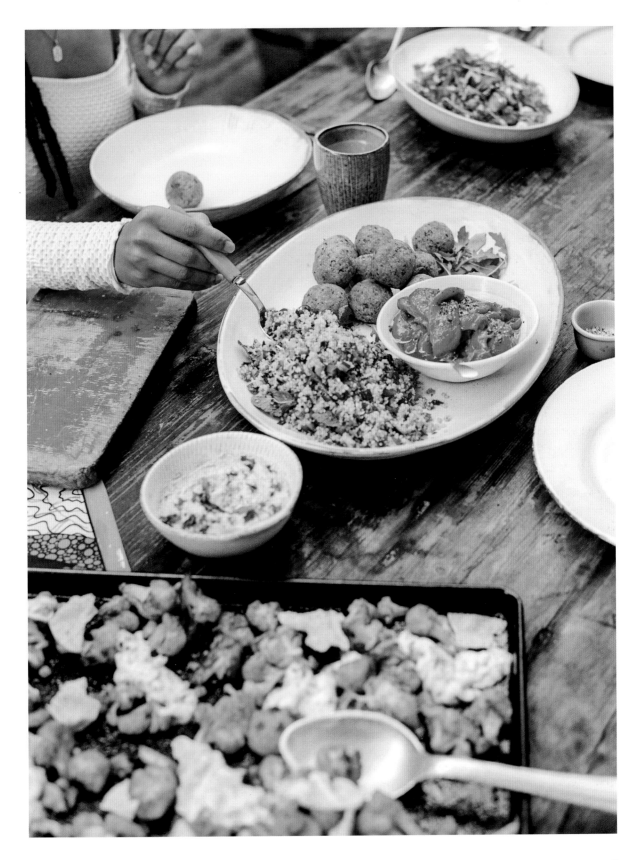

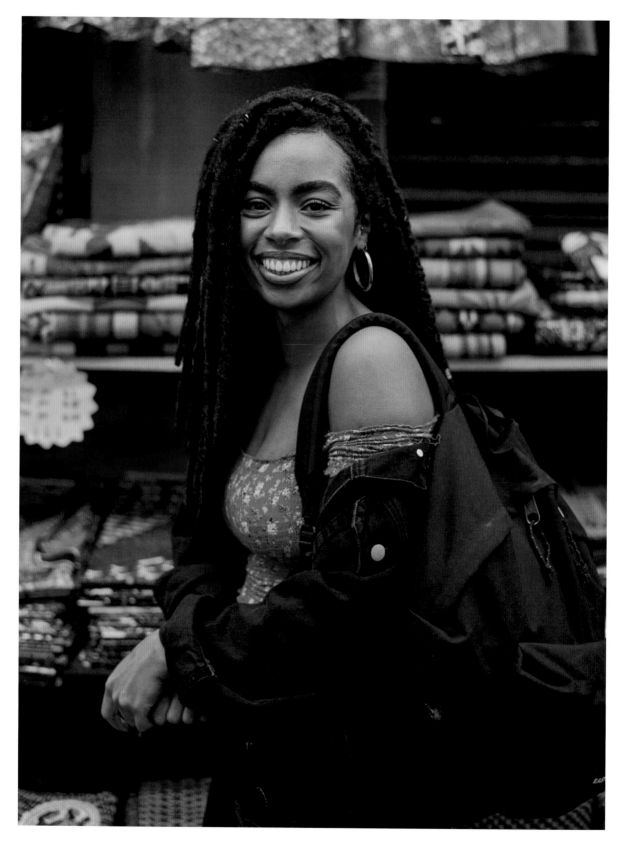

Introduction

more about them and why I like using them. Don't worry, there are lots of simple recipes with ingredients you can get at your standard supermarket!

If you have seen my YouTube channel or Instagram, you'll know about my love for music and dance. I grew up in a household where music was always playing; my brother even started producing his own music before he got into his current career. And when I wasn't playing football I was also in a dance troupe performing in shows from when I was seven until my late teens. I had to infuse this love of music and dance in the book so I've listed songs for some of the recipes! It's not essential to listen to them but if you want to hear a few tunes while you cook, these are some suggestions. When I'm cooking there is always a DJ set going on to sing and dance to. I love a two-step to cook to, so most are two-step friendly. There are some old-school tunes, some new, some reggae, some neo-soul – there is a real variety and to listen to the entire selection back to back as a playlist would probably sound very random as some are matched to cuisines too. I probably know the lyrics to almost all the tracks as there have been times in my life when I've played them on repeat. For example, 'We Are One' by Maze feat. Frankie Beverly (see page 199) reminds me of summers in Barbados when I was growing up and my mum's friends would throw raves and end the night singing their hearts out and two-stepping to this classic. 'Dance Tonight' by Lucy Pearl (see page 149) is the sound of summer barbecues, every time! 'One Night Only' by Mahalia feat. Kojey Radical – I'm in the music video! 'This Is How We Do It' by Montell Jordan (see page 136) reminds me of a dance show I was in when I was about 12. And 'Chan Chan' by Buena Vista Social Club (see page 143) is one of my favourite songs of all time. I could really go on about each song but I won't bore you with that!

This book comes straight from my heart direct to your plate, and hopefully to your soul too. I hope it fills you up and inspires many more flavourful meals and recipes from plants!

I love seeing what you're eating so please do share your recreations with me by tagging me on Instagram @rachelama_ and don't forget to have fun and, of course, two-step!

Love, Rach xx

1

BREAKFAST AND BRUNCH

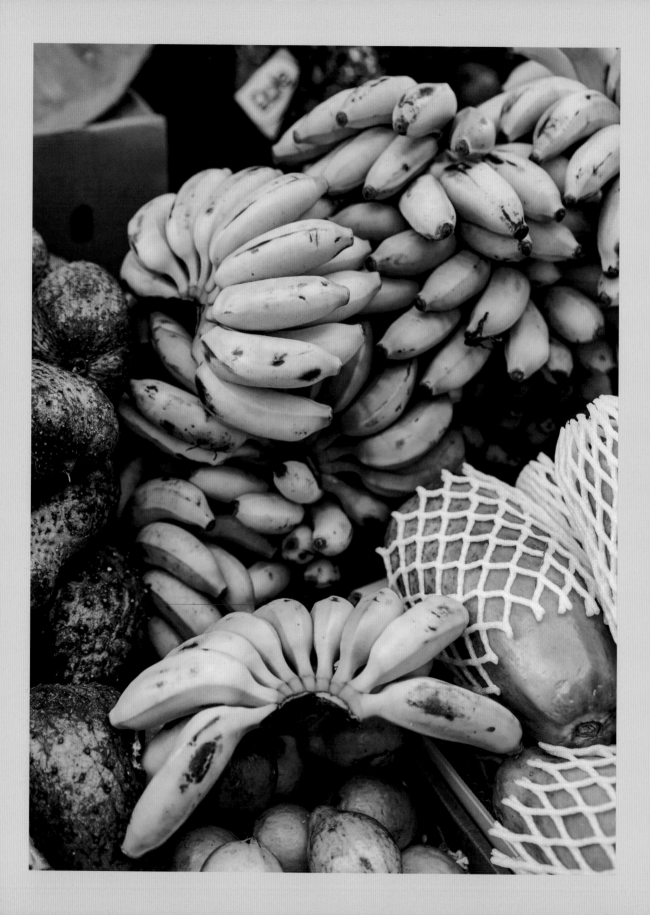

Breakfast and Brunch

Breakfast is a really important meal for me. It's how I ensure I start the day right, with some good fuel and energy, especially knowing that once I leave the house there is a good chance it will be a little difficult finding a good, quick vegan meal out and about. A proper breakfast is the best way to avoid a hangry Rachel.

My go-to breakfast for busy days is a very easy porridge; I just jazz it up depending on what season it is and what fruits, seeds and nuts I'm feeling. But there are so many different breakfast and brunch recipes that you can make.

In this chapter you'll find savoury waffles, one-pan breakfasts, sweet pancakes, breakfast burritos and ackee scramble bagels – a real variety of options to choose from to keep your plant-based breakfasts exciting. Some recipes you'll be able to make ahead for those busy weekdays when you don't have time in the morning, some are quick and easy, and some require a little more time but are well worth that extra effort for a delicious feast at the weekend.

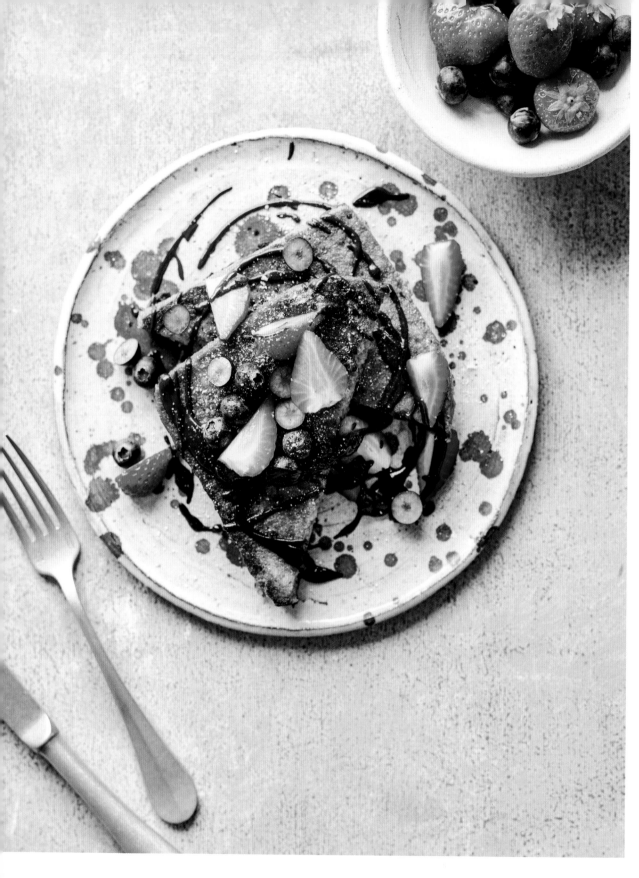

Breakfast and Brunch

Serves 4

8 thick slices of
   sourdough bread
Coconut oil, for frying

For the chocolate sauce
180g vegan dark chocolate,
   broken into squares
1–2 tbsp coconut oil
1 tbsp maple syrup

For the French toast batter
2 tsp vanilla extract
4 tbsp chickpea flour
120ml plant-based milk
   (to make your own,
   see page 238)
1 tsp ground cinnamon
2 tbsp maple syrup
Pinch of salt

To serve
75g blueberries
75g strawberries, hulled
   and sliced lengthways
Icing sugar, for dusting

Cinnamon French Toast Drizzled in Chocolate

One of the best ways to turn a stale end-of-week loaf into a perfect Saturday morning treat. The chickpea batter gently softens the bread while the maple syrup makes the outside lightly crisp and caramelised as it cooks. I love this with fresh berries and lots of chocolate drizzled all over, but you can substitute the chocolate for a generous drizzle of maple syrup if you don't have chocolate on the mind as much as I do.

First make the chocolate sauce. Fill a saucepan with water to a depth of 2–3cm and bring to a simmer, then reduce the heat to low. Place the chocolate in a heatproof bowl that will fit snugly on top of the pan without the simmering water touching the base of the bowl. Stir the chocolate occasionally as it begins to soften, then add 1 tablespoon of the coconut oil and the maple syrup. Add more coconut oil, 1 teaspoon at a time, if the mixture is still too thick. Remove the pan from the heat once the chocolate has melted and set aside.

Meanwhile, place all the ingredients for the French toast batter into a bowl – one that is wide enough to soak a slice of bread – and whisk together until smooth.

Add one slice of bread to the mixture and leave for a few seconds to soak in the batter before turning, so that both sides are evenly coated.

Melt 1 tablespoon of coconut oil in a frying pan over a gentle heat. Once melted, add the batter-soaked bread to the pan and cook for about 7 minutes until browned before turning over and cooking for another 3–4 minutes on the other side. Continue to soak and cook the remaining slices of bread, using more coconut oil as needed. As you fry each slice of bread, keep the rest warm on a baking sheet in the oven on a low heat.

Divide the French toast between plates and sprinkle over a handful of blueberries and sliced strawberries, then drizzle over the melted chocolate and dust with icing sugar to serve.

Serves 1

2 slices of sourdough bread
1 tbsp maple syrup

For the toppings

**Peanut butter, banana
and hemp seeds**
2 tbsp peanut butter
    (to make your own,
    see page 240)
1 banana, sliced
1 tbsp hemp seeds

**Peanut butter, chia jam
and coconut flakes**
2 tbsp peanut butter
    (to make your own,
    see page 240)
80g Chia Raspberry Jam
    (see page 35)
1 tbsp coconut flakes

**Almond butter, blueberries
and cocoa nibs**
2 tbsp almond butter
    (to make your own,
    see page 240)
75g blueberries
1 tbsp cocoa nibs
1 tbsp hemp seeds

**Almond butter, apples,
cinnamon and hemp seeds**
2 tbsp almond butter
    (to make your own,
    see page 240)
1 apple, peeled and sliced
1 tsp ground cinnamon
1 tbsp pecans
1 tbsp hemp seeds

Nut Butter Toast Galore

The perfect quick snack. Sourdough toast
spread with nut butter and sprinkled with your
favourite fruits or nuts and a drizzle of maple
syrup – so simple and quick, yet so, so delicious!

Toast the bread and spread with nut butter.

Add one of the toppings and drizzle with maple syrup.

TOM MISCH - 'SUNSHINE'

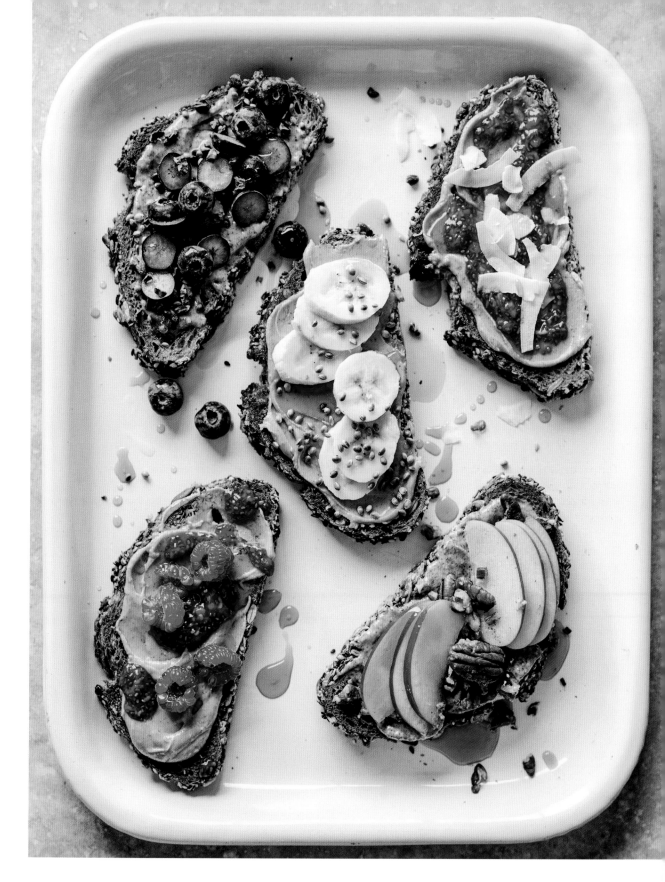

Serves 1

For the smoothie
4 ice cubes
120–160ml plant-based milk
    (to make your own,
    see page 238)
1 tbsp açai powder
25g rolled oats
1 scoop of protein powder
    (following packet
    instructions for
    dosage; optional)
2 dates, pitted
    (or 2 tbsp maple syrup)
1 tbsp chia seeds
150–180g frozen
    mixed berries

To serve
1 banana, sliced
30g Granola (see page 25)
1 tbsp hemp seeds
40g raspberries
1 tbsp coconut flakes

Berry Smoothie Bowl

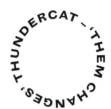

A quick and easy mixed berry bowl! I love making these in the summertime after a workout, to cool myself down in the sun, with a scoop of protein powder to help replenish my energy. I became obsessed with açai bowls from my time in Brazil in 2015, but found it hard to get hold of fresh açai purée without added sugars in the UK, so I began whizzing together frozen berries with pure açai powder for a similar effect. It creates this deliciously thick and smooth mixture, to which you can add dates for a bit of sweetness and top with fresh fruit and coconut flakes.

Place all the smoothie ingredients in a high-speed blender or food processor and mix until smooth. For a thicker consistency, use the larger quantity of frozen berries, or for a runnier consistency, use the larger amount of milk.

Pour the mixture into a bowl and top with the banana, granola, hemp seeds, raspberries and coconut flakes.

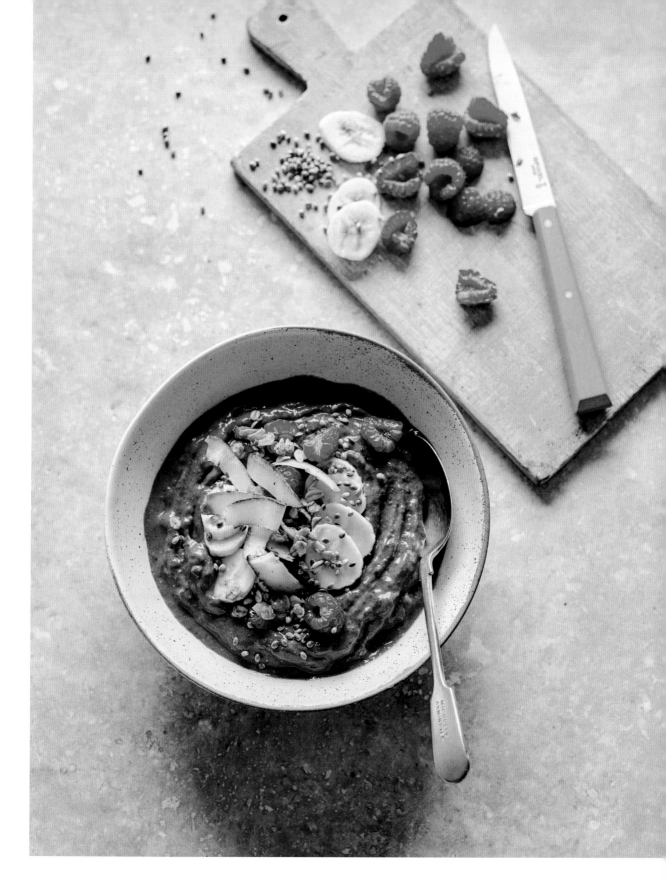

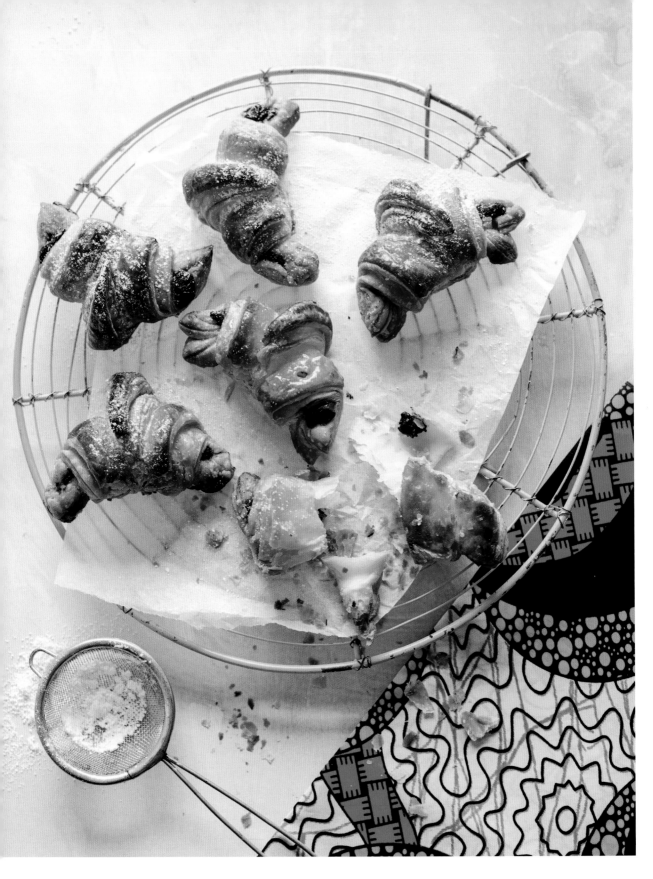

Breakfast and Brunch

Makes 6 croissants

2 tbsp vegan butter, plus
    extra for greasing
Plain flour, for dusting
320g ready-rolled puff pastry
    sheet (I use Jus-Rol)
50g vegan dark chocolate

60ml plant-based milk
    (to make your own,
    see page 238)
2 tbsp maple syrup, plus an
    optional extra tablespoon
Icing sugar (optional)

Quick Mini Chocolate Croissants

I didn't really think I'd get to eat croissants again when I first went vegan, plus the French pâtisserie classic does require some serious skill if you make it yourself. These delicious bite-sized chocolate croissants are an amazing super-simple alternative. They're perfect as a morning snack, especially if you're hosting a brunch for friends. You can make them without the chocolate; just serve them plain with jam instead or your favourite sweet fillings. You can also make them savoury by slicing the croissants in half and putting vegan cheese and sliced tomatoes inside.

Preheat the oven to 180°C fan (or following the packet instructions for cooking the puff pastry). Line a baking sheet with baking paper or grease with butter.

On a work surface lightly dusted with flour, unfold the pastry sheet and use a rolling pin to roll the sheet until the long side of the rectangle has doubled in length – keep the shape by rolling it from the short ends.

Spread 1 tablespoon of the butter across half of the rolled-out pastry sheet and then fold it in half widthways. Lightly roll out the pastry again widthways, keeping the rectangular shape, to seal the butter, then spread the rest of the butter over the top of the pastry in a thin layer.

Along the top of the long side of the rectangle, measure and mark 10cm intervals then, using a sharp knife, slice in a diagonal line from the first interval on the left down to the left-hand corner on the bottom edge of the rectangle to create a triangle. Do the same on the right. Now measure 10cm in from the bottom edge of the rectangle and cut a diagonal slice up to the top left corner to create another triangle. Repeat until you have six triangles.

Continued on the next page

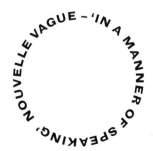

NOUVELLE VAGUE – 'IN A MANNER OF SPEAKING'

Cut the chocolate into thin rectangles – about 1cm wide by 2–3cm long – and place two in the middle of each triangle. Then, starting at the base of the triangle, roll up each triangle to enclose the chocolate. Place each croissant with the tip of the triangle facing upwards, then gently pinch the edges round to create a croissant shape and place on the prepared baking sheet.

Mix the milk with the maple syrup and then brush each croissant with this mixture. Place in the oven to bake for about 25 minutes or until the croissants are puffed up and golden brown.

Allow the croissants to cool down a little, as the melted chocolate will be very hot, then transfer to a plate and serve with a dusting of icing sugar for a professional finish, or brush the tops of the croissants with the extra tablespoon of maple syrup for a glossy glazed finish.

Makes about 1.35kg

500g mixed nuts (such as almonds, Brazil nuts, walnuts, cashews and hazelnuts)

250g pecans

125g macadamia nuts

100g sunflower seeds

125g pumpkin seeds

250g rolled oats

3 tbsp coconut oil, melted

4–5 tbsp maple syrup

2 tsp ground cinnamon

Granola

I can't get enough of this granola! It is an everyday essential in my house – every 6 weeks or so, I make a big batch. Sweetened with just a touch of maple syrup, this is guaranteed to make your house smell amazing as it cooks. You can add a bit of dried fruit at the end, if you like, such as raisins or dried apricots. I've played around with different amounts of coconut oil for crunch and maple syrup for sweetness to get it the way I like it. I keep it simple and nutty with just a little sweetness but not too much as more maple syrup can be added when you serve it, if need be. The more you make home-made granola, the more you can adjust the ingredients to your preference.

Preheat the oven to 180°C fan.

Place all the nuts in a food processor and pulse to break them down slightly. I like to keep mine relatively chunky so I don't pulse them too much.

Tip the nuts into a large bowl and mix in the sunflower and pumpkin seeds and the oats. Pour in the coconut oil and 3 tablespoons of the maple syrup, add the cinnamon and mix in well. Taste and add more maple syrup, if needed, though you'll need to keep an eye on the mixture as it cooks to prevent it burning.

Spread the granola out evenly on a baking tray – use two trays if necessary. Place in the oven to bake for 20 minutes, then remove from the oven to give the mixture a good stir before baking for another 15 minutes or until roasted and golden. Check every so often to ensure that the granola isn't browning too quickly. Stir the mixture again if it is, and take out of the oven earlier, if needed.

Remove from the oven and allow to cool completely before storing in an airtight container for up to 2 months.

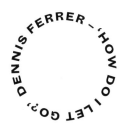

DENNIS FERRER – 'HOW DO I LET GO?'

160g quinoa flour
1 tsp baking powder
½ tsp bicarbonate of soda
1 tbsp chia seeds
250ml plant-based milk
(to make your own,
see page 238)
1 tsp apple cider vinegar
1 tbsp maple syrup, plus
extra for drizzling
75g blueberries,
plus extra to serve
Coconut oil, for frying

**For the whipped
coconut cream**
1 × 400ml tin of full-fat
coconut milk
1 tbsp maple syrup
Pinch of finely grated
lemon zest

Fluffy Berry Quinoa Pancakes

These little pancakes made from quinoa flour are amazing! Quinoa flour is so nutritious, and adding omega-rich chia seeds and juicy blueberries makes these pancakes light and fluffy and incredibly filling. Drizzled in maple syrup and served with a delicious whipped coconut cream, they are a real delight. For ease and to save time, you could use a shop-bought coconut cream for the topping instead, if you prefer.

To make the whipped coconut cream, place the tin of coconut milk in the fridge overnight, or for at least 12 hours. Chilling the milk will encourage the coconut water to separate from the thick cream.

The next day, open the tin and carefully tip out the water, reserving it to use in smoothies or juices. Scoop the leftover thick coconut cream into a bowl and whisk using an electric hand whisk for a few minutes. You can whisk it by hand but it will take a bit longer – up to 15 minutes. Add the maple syrup and lemon zest and whisk for another minute or so, until the cream is whipped to your liking.

For the pancakes, start by sifting the flour, baking powder and bicarbonate of soda into a large bowl, then mix in the chia seeds. Add the milk, followed by the apple cider vinegar and maple syrup, then mix everything together well to combine all the ingredients. Carefully fold in the blueberries.

Melt 1 tablespoon of coconut oil in a large non-stick frying pan over a gentle heat. Add roughly 60ml of the batter to the pan for one pancake. (Depending on the size of your pan, you may be able to cook more than one pancake at a time.) Let this cook for about 4 minutes until holes begin to appear in the surface of the pancake and you can easily slide a spatula underneath. Flip over, and cook for another 2–3 minutes on the other side.

Repeat until all the batter is used up, using more coconut oil as needed. If not serving the pancakes immediately, keep them warm on a baking sheet in the oven on a low heat.

Divide between plates and serve topped with extra blueberries, maple syrup and a dollop of whipped coconut cream.

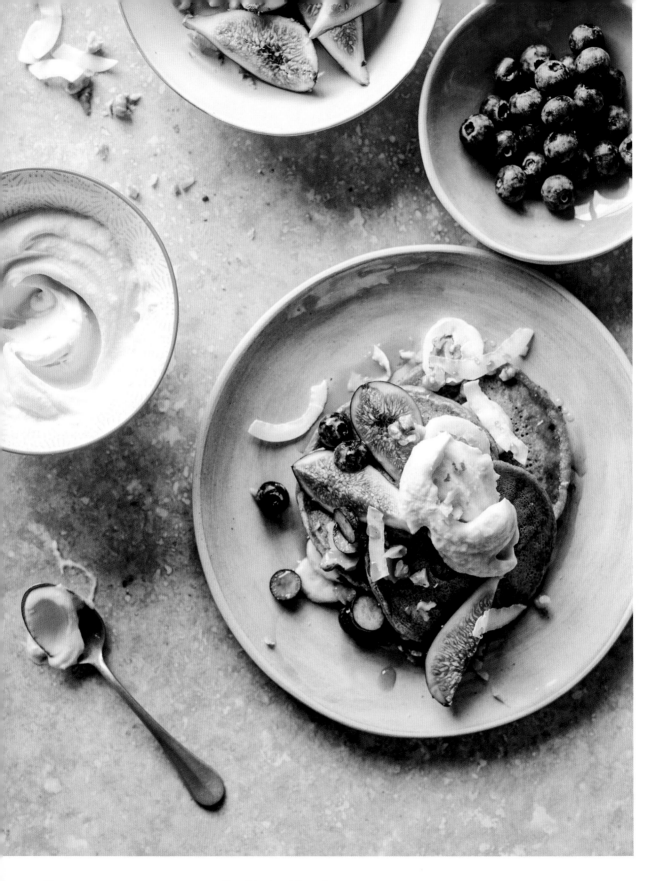

Breakfast and Brunch

Makes 8 pancakes

125g plain flour
1 tbsp baking powder
1 tbsp moringa powder
Pinch of salt
240ml plant-based milk
  (to make your own,
  see page 238)
1 tbsp fresh lemon juice
1 tsp vanilla extract
1 tbsp maple syrup
Coconut oil, for frying

To serve
125g walnuts, lightly crushed
2 tbsp coconut flakes
4 fresh figs, roughly chopped
3 bananas, sliced
Handful of blueberries
1 quantity of Whipped
  Coconut Cream
  (see page 26)
60ml maple syrup or Toffee
  Sauce (see page 223)

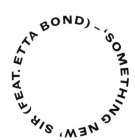

Moringa Pancakes with Figs and Walnuts

Don't be scared by the green colour! These delicious fluffy pancakes, topped with crunchy walnuts, fresh blueberries, sliced bananas and whipped coconut cream, are so tasty. One way I sometimes add extra nutrients to my pancakes is by stirring in a powder, like moringa, which is why these are green. It doesn't add much taste but if it's not your thing, feel free to leave it out.

Sift the flour, baking powder, moringa powder and salt into a large bowl. In a separate bowl, mix together the milk, lemon juice, vanilla extract and maple syrup and set aside to rest for 5 minutes.

Pour the wet mixture into the bowl with the dry ingredients and whisk until smooth.

Melt 1 tablespoon of coconut oil in a non-stick frying pan over a medium heat. Add roughly 4 tablespoons of the batter to the pan for one pancake. (Depending on the size of your pan, you may be able to cook more than one pancake at a time.) Let this cook for about 4 minutes until holes begin to appear in the surface and you can easily slide a spatula underneath. Flip it over, and cook for another 2–3 minutes on the other side.

Repeat until all the batter is used up, using more coconut oil as needed. If not serving the pancakes immediately, keep them warm on a baking sheet in the oven on a low heat.

Divide the pancakes between plates and top with the walnuts, coconut flakes, figs, bananas and blueberries. Add a dollop of the whipped coconut cream and drizzle with maple syrup or toffee sauce.

Makes 12–14 pancakes

2 ripe bananas, peeled
270g rolled oats,
    plus more if needed
480ml plant-based milk
    (to make your own,
    see page 238)
Coconut oil, for frying

To serve
1 quantity of Chia Raspberry
    Jam (see page 35)
1 quantity of Whipped
    Coconut Cream
    (see page 26)
2 tbsp maple syrup

Three-ingredient Pancakes

The easiest pancakes to make, with just three simple ingredients. Nutritious oats are a great way to start the day, so why not turn them into delicious pancakes? When I first went vegan, I made these all of the time as they're so versatile. Here they're topped with home-made chia jam and whipped coconut cream, but you could substitute with any of your favourite toppings or add raw cacao to the batter to turn them into chocolate pancakes (about 2–3 tablespoons, depending on how chocolatey you want them).

Place the bananas, rolled oats and milk in a blender or food processor and blend together. The batter should be relatively thick. If it seems too thin and runny, add more oats, 1 tablespoon at a time, to thicken it slightly.

Melt 1 tablespoon of coconut oil in a large non-stick frying pan set over a gentle heat. Add roughly 4 tablespoons of the batter to the pan for one pancake. (Depending on the size of your pan, you may be able to cook more than one pancake at a time.) Let this cook for about 2 minutes until holes begin to appear in the surface of the pancake and you can easily slide a spatula underneath. Flip it over, and cook for another 2 minutes on the other side.

Repeat until all the batter is used up, using more coconut oil as needed. If not serving the pancakes immediately, keep them warm on a baking sheet in the oven on a low heat.

Divide the pancakes between plates and drizzle with the chia jam, add a large spoonful of whipped coconut cream and then drizzle over the maple syrup.

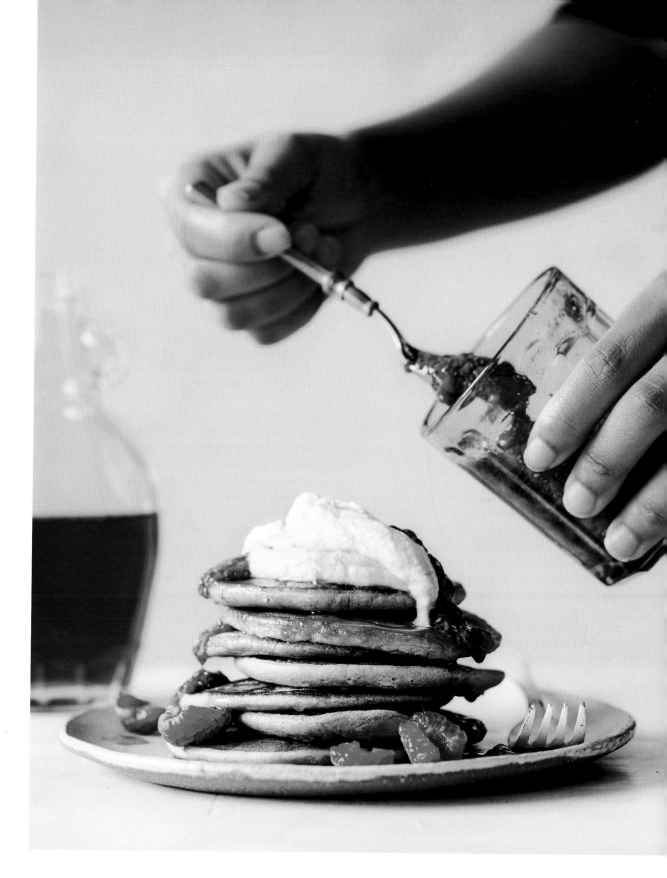

For the chia pudding
720ml coconut milk
8 tbsp chia seeds
1 tbsp vanilla extract
60ml maple syrup
Pinch of salt

For the mango purée
1 ripe mango
1 tbsp fresh lemon juice
1 tbsp maple syrup (optional, for sweetness)
2 tbsp water (optional)

To serve
2 tbsp coconut flakes
100g Granola (see page 25)

You will need
4 cups or jars

Coconut Vanilla Chia Pudding with Mango Purée

Chia seeds are everything to me, I think they play a large part in keeping my digestion healthy. I personally love the texture: they absorb liquid and become soft and silky and go so well with the mango. Make these ahead and chill them overnight to start your day with a yummy tropical pudding!

To make the chia pudding, pour the coconut milk into a bowl, or a container with a lid, and add the chia seeds, vanilla extract, maple syrup and salt. Mix until well combined, then cover with a plate, or the container lid, and place in the fridge to set overnight or for a minimum of 2 hours.

Meanwhile, peel and dice the mango into small chunks, then place in a blender or food processor with the lemon juice and the maple syrup, if needed, and blend to a purée. If the mango seems a bit dry, add the water to help blend it to a purée. For an even smoother texture, push the purée through a fine sieve.

Once the chia pudding has set, place a generous layer into each of the cups or jars, followed by a layer of mango purée, then add another generous portion of chia pudding. Top with more mango purée and sprinkle with the coconut flakes and granola to serve.

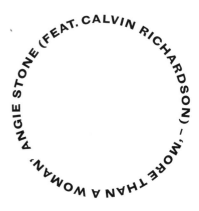
ANGIE STONE (FEAT. CALVIN RICHARDSON) – 'MORE THAN A WOMAN,'

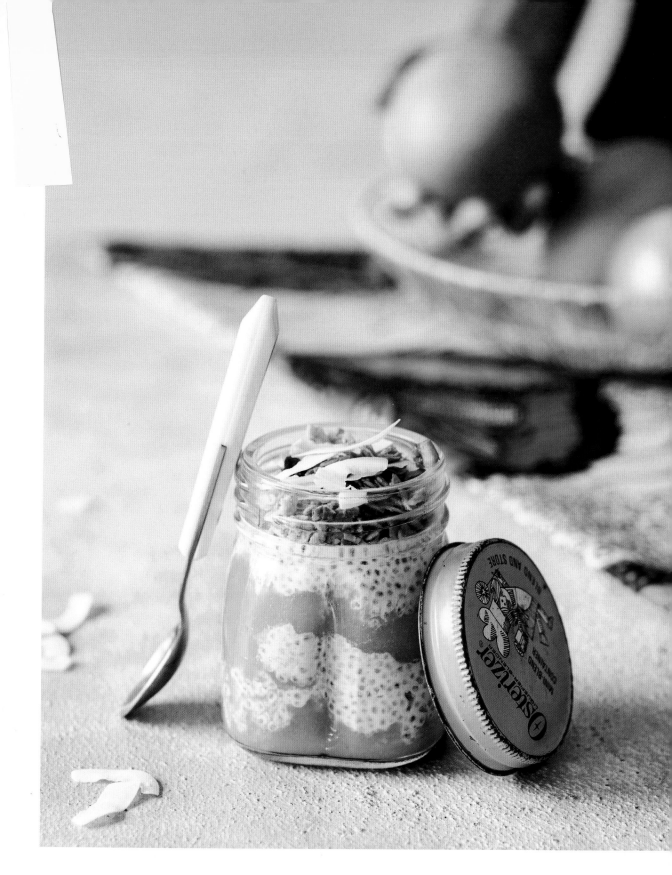

160g rolled oats

480–720ml plant-based milk
(to make your own,
see page 238)

60ml maple syrup

2 tsp ground cinnamon
(optional)

4 tbsp chia seeds

To serve

75g blueberries

4 bananas, sliced

200g Granola
(see page 25)

Porridge

My favourite go-to breakfast to start the day. Creamy oats and chia seeds topped with blueberries, sliced bananas and home-made granola. Simple, delicious and versatile. In the summer I love to top my porridge with a variety of fresh fruits, while in the winter I warm up a handful of frozen mixed berries and sprinkle them on top with the granola and a drizzle of maple syrup – an instant berry-like crumble, and so luscious! I have this breakfast nearly every day in the week, I just switch up the fruits from time to time. When I want a quick chocolate fix – quite often – I love to add raw cacao powder to the porridge; it's like a hot chocolate porridge, so comforting!

Place the oats in a medium saucepan and pour in 480ml of the milk. Stir in the maple syrup and cinnamon (if using). Bring to the boil, then reduce the heat and simmer for 4 minutes, stirring occasionally to ensure the porridge does not stick to the base of the pan.

Remove from the heat and mix in the chia seeds. You can add the rest of the milk if you prefer a runnier porridge.

Pour the porridge into bowls and top each with a few blueberries, sliced bananas and a handful of granola.

CHOCOLATE PORRIDGE

For chocolate porridge, add 4 tablespoons of raw cacao powder to the pan with the maple syrup, cinnamon (if using) and a small pinch of salt, and then make the porridge as above.

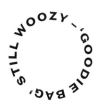

'STILL WOOZY – 'GOODIE BAG'

Makes 4 pots

180g rolled oats
480ml plant-based milk
    (to make your own,
    see page 238)
300ml vegan cream
2 tbsp maple syrup
125g smooth natural peanut
    butter (to make your own,
    see page 240)

For the chia raspberry jam

300g frozen raspberries
120ml water
2–3 tbsp maple syrup
2 tbsp chia seeds

To serve

2 bananas, sliced
120g Granola (see page 25)

You will need
4 lidded pots or jars

Overnight Peanut Butter and Chia Jam Oats

Creamy oats with a peanut butter and chia jam twist. Perfect to make ahead for breakfast the next day.

Place the oats in a large bowl, add the milk, cream, maple syrup and peanut butter and mix together well, then set aside while you make the chia raspberry jam.

Place the raspberries and water in a saucepan, add 2 tablespoons of the maple syrup and cook over a low heat for a few minutes until the berries have softened. Using the back of a spatula, gently push down on the berries to create a more jam-like texture.

Remove from the heat and add the chia seeds. Mix in well and leave to sit for about 5 minutes until the chia seeds expand and the jam thickens. Taste and add more maple syrup, if needed.

Place a layer of soaked oats into each of the pots or jars, followed by a layer of chia jam, then another layer each of oats and jam. Close each pot/jar with a lid and chill in the fridge overnight or for a minimum of 2 hours. Top each pot with banana slices and granola to serve.

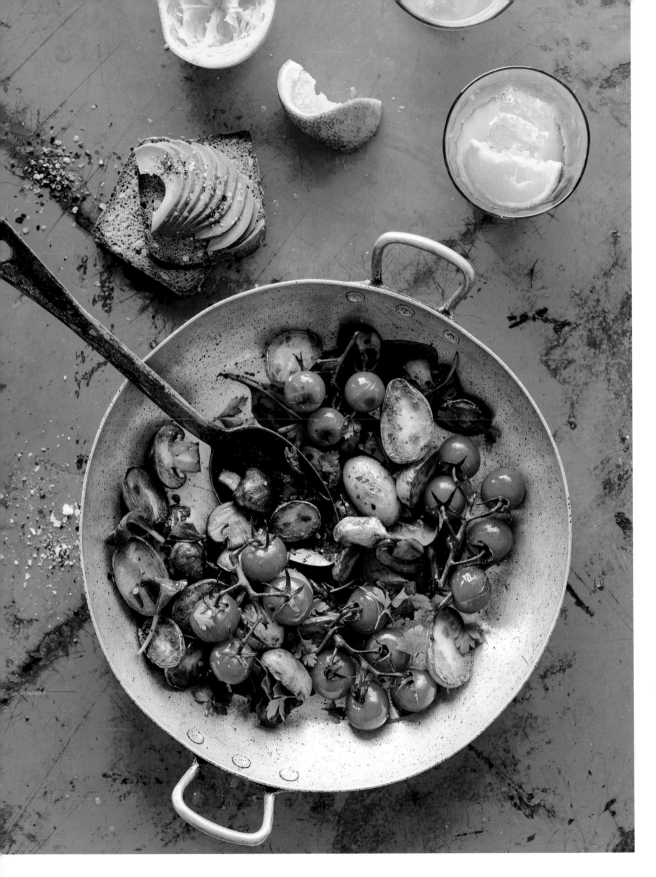

Breakfast and Brunch

Serves 2

1–2 tbsp olive oil

4 baby new potatoes
(unpeeled), halved
or quartered

Handful of cherry
tomatoes on the vine

1 garlic clove, thinly sliced

Handful of chestnut
mushrooms, halved

Large handful of spinach

Small handful of parsley,
roughly chopped, plus
extra to serve

Salt and black pepper

To serve

½ avocado, sliced

Chilli flakes, for sprinkling
(optional)

One-pan Breakfast

Crispy new potatoes with cherry tomatoes, garlic mushrooms and spinach all cooked in one pan. A savoury start to the day that requires minimal washing up. If I've got a long day ahead of me sometimes I mix it up and add some beans to make it even more filling.

Pour the olive oil into a frying pan, add the potatoes and fry over a medium heat for 5–7 minutes until starting to brown and soften slightly, then move the potatoes to one side, turn up the heat a little and add the tomatoes, garlic and mushrooms and fry until everything is cooked through and golden.

Add the spinach and chopped parsley, stirring it in until wilted, season to taste with salt and pepper and then remove from the heat.

Top with the avocado and sprinkle with chilli flakes (if using) and a little more parsley to serve.

Serves 4

4 bagels, halved
2 avocados, sliced
1 quantity of Smoky
    Aubergine (see page 46)
4 tbsp pumpkin seeds
1 tbsp finely snipped chives
Handful of fresh coriander,
    chopped
1 lime, cut into 4 wedges,
    to serve

For the ackee scramble

1 tbsp vegetable oil
1 onion, finely chopped
2 spring onions,
    finely chopped
3 garlic cloves,
    finely chopped
Leaves from 2 thyme sprigs
1 tsp ground turmeric
2 plum tomatoes,
    roughly chopped
1 small fresh red chilli,
    deseeded and
    finely chopped
1 tbsp nutritional yeast
1 × 540g tin of ackee, drained
1 tbsp fresh lime juice
Salt (or black salt)
    and black pepper

Ackee Scramble and Smoky Aubergine Bagels

A mouth-watering vegan take on a breakfast classic, a savoury mixture of onions, tomatoes and ackee – one of my favourite natural alternatives to eggs. Ackee is a fruit that you'll see in a lot of Caribbean cooking. It's extremely subtle in taste and soaks up flavour well, just be careful not to over-mix it as it breaks down very easily. The aim is to heat it up and give it just a few stirs when cooking. Using black salt to season the ackee right at the end of cooking will give an egg-like flavour to this dish, which is really delicious. I've topped the ackee with sweet and smoky, slightly crispy aubergines and served them in a toasted bagel with some avocado for ultimate bagel goals.

Preheat the oven to 180°C fan.

First make the ackee scramble. Place the vegetable oil in a medium saucepan over a medium heat, add the onion and spring onions and sauté for 5 minutes until softened, then add the garlic, thyme, turmeric, tomatoes and chilli, season with pepper and sauté for a further 5 minutes.

Sprinkle in the nutritional yeast and then add the ackee. Give this a gentle mix to coat the ackee in all the other ingredients and then allow to heat through for 4–5 minutes. Ackee is fragile so don't over-mix or it will turn to mush.

Remove from the heat, add the lime juice and ½ teaspoon of salt and mix in carefully.

Meanwhile, toast the bagel halves and place two halves on each plate.

Add some of the ackee scramble to the bottom half of each bagel, along with a few slices of avocado and smoky aubergine, then sprinkle with pumpkin seeds, chives and coriander before adding the top half of the bagel. Serve each filled bagel with a wedge of lime for squeezing over.

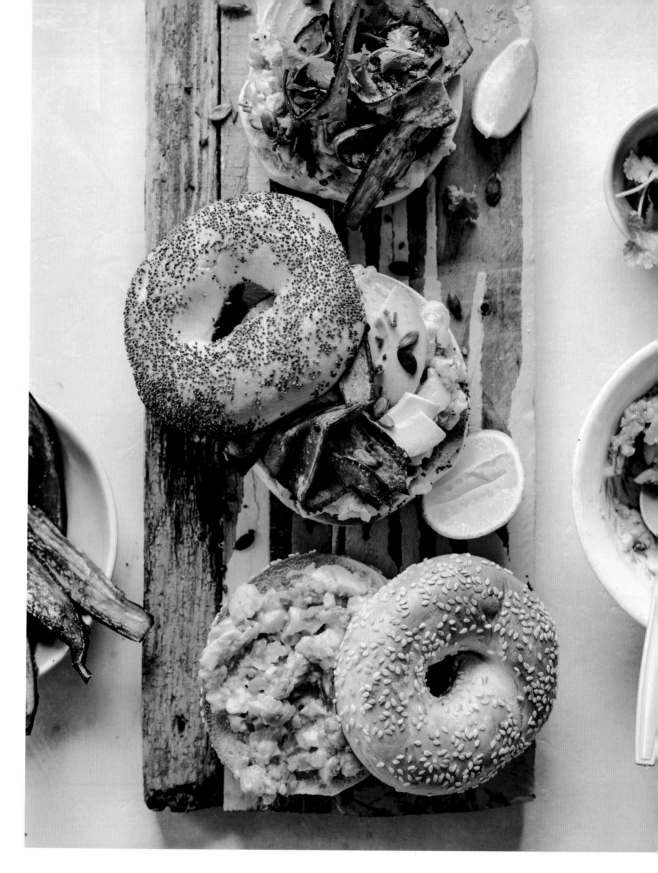

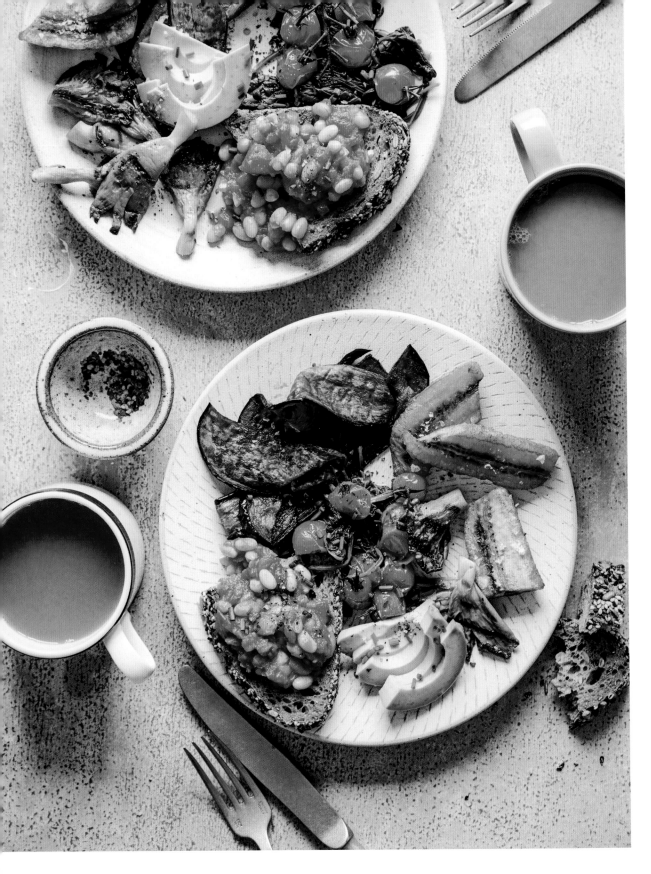

Breakfast and Brunch

Serves 4

8 slices of seeded
    sourdough bread
55g vegan butter
1 quantity of Smoky
    Aubergine (see page 46)
1 quantity of Tomatoes and
    Spinach (see page 43)
½ quantity of Fried Plantains
    (see page 174)
2 avocados, sliced
Chilli flakes, for sprinkling
1 tbsp snipped chives

For the baked beans

1 tbsp vegetable oil
1 white onion, finely chopped
4 garlic cloves, finely chopped
2 × 400g tins of chopped
    tomatoes
2 × 400g tins of haricot
    beans, drained and rinsed
1 tbsp balsamic vinegar
1 tsp vegan
    Worcestershire sauce
1 tbsp soy sauce
    (or coconut aminos)
1 tbsp maple syrup
Salt and black pepper

For the mushrooms

375g oyster mushrooms,
    roughly chopped
1 tbsp liquid smoke (or soy
    sauce or coconut aminos)
1 tbsp soy sauce
    (or coconut aminos)
1 tsp chilli flakes
1 tbsp vegetable oil
1 tbsp chopped parsley

Vegan Full English Breakfast

Served with a reviving cup of tea, this vegan take on a British classic is what Sunday mornings were made for! An unbeatable mixture of delicious home-made baked beans, sweet and smoky aubergines, velvety mushrooms, juicy cherry tomatoes, spinach and fried plantain. When I was growing up, my grandma used to cook plantains and bacon for us, so naturally plantains became a staple part of my very English breakfasts!

First make the baked beans. Place the vegetable oil in a large saucepan, add the onion and garlic, season with salt and pepper and sauté over a medium heat for 5–6 minutes until softened. Pour in the tinned tomatoes and haricot beans, followed by the balsamic vinegar, Worcestershire sauce, soy sauce and maple syrup. Stir together well and cook on a low heat for about 7 minutes.

Meanwhile, place the mushrooms in a bowl with the liquid smoke, soy sauce and chilli flakes, season with salt and pepper and mix until the mushrooms are evenly coated.

Place the vegetable oil in a frying pan or griddle pan set over a gentle heat and add the soy-coated mushrooms. Cook for 5–6 minutes, stirring occasionally, until browned and any liquid has evaporated. Once cooked, sprinkle with the parsley.

Toast the sourdough bread and spread each slice with butter. To each plate add two slices of buttered toast and a portion of baked beans, smoky aubergine, fried mushrooms, tomatoes and spinach, fried plantains and avocado, then sprinkle with chilli flakes and chives and finish with a grind of pepper.

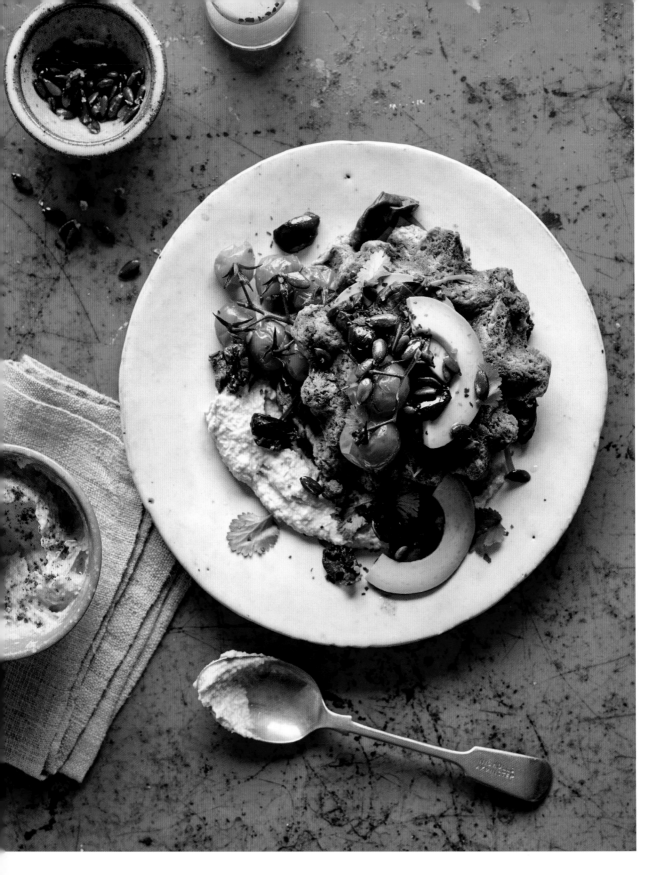

Breakfast and Brunch

Makes 4–6 waffles

1 quantity of Hummus
   (see page 177)
2 avocados, sliced
2 tbsp extra-virgin olive oil
Juice of 1 lemon
Handful of fresh coriander,
   chopped
2 tbsp pumpkin seeds
100g pitted mixed olives,
   sliced
1 tbsp chilli flakes

For the waffles
3 spring onions, chopped
2 garlic cloves, chopped
2 tbsp fresh lemon juice
15g fresh coriander,
   roughly chopped
15g fresh parsley,
   roughly chopped
½ tsp ground cumin
¼ tsp ground coriander
½ tsp paprika
½ tsp cayenne pepper
1 tbsp nutritional yeast
1 × 400g tin of chickpeas,
   drained and rinsed
150g plain flour

1 tbsp baking powder
1 tsp bicarbonate of soda
240ml plant-based milk
   (to make your own,
   see page 238)
1 tsp apple cider vinegar
6 tbsp rapeseed oil
Salt and black pepper

**For the tomatoes
and spinach**
360g cherry tomatoes
   on the vine
200g spinach

You will need a waffle iron

Spiced Chickpea Waffles

Infused with delicious East African spices, these waffles are really tasty and their texture is perfect: a little crispy on the outside and soft inside. A super-filling breakfast or lunch, you can even make them ahead and lightly toast them later in the day for a snack topped with hummus and avocado.

Heat a waffle iron.

Place all the waffle ingredients, except the flour, baking powder, bicarbonate of soda, milk, apple cider vinegar and oil in a blender or food processor, season with a teaspoon of salt and pepper to taste and pulse to break down the chickpeas slightly and combine the ingredients.

Put the flour into a large bowl and stir in the baking powder and bicarbonate of soda, then pour in the chickpea mixture followed by the milk, apple cider vinegar and oil. Mix well to combine.

Add roughly 2 large tablespoons of the mixture per waffle to the waffle iron. Cook for about 10 minutes, or according to the manufacturer's instructions, until the outside has browned.

Meanwhile, place the cherry tomatoes in a medium saucepan (removing them from the vine first, if you prefer) and season with salt and pepper. Cover with a lid and cook for 10 minutes on a low heat until tender, then tip in the spinach, season again with salt and pepper and cook until the spinach is slightly wilted.

Place a waffle on each plate and add a generous spoonful of hummus, followed by the cooked tomatoes and spinach and some sliced avocado. Drizzle with olive oil and a squeeze of lemon juice and sprinkle with the coriander, pumpkin seeds, olives and chilli flakes.

Serves 4

4 large soft flour tortillas
200g spinach
1 quantity of Guacamole
(see page 180)
1 quantity of Cherry Tomato
Salsa (see page 182)
1 lime, cut into 4 wedges
Handful of fresh coriander,
chopped

For the chickpea scramble
1 tbsp olive oil
1 red onion, finely sliced
1 red pepper, deseeded
and diced
2 × 400g tins of chickpeas,
drained and rinsed
3 garlic cloves,
finely chopped

2 tsp ground turmeric
2 tsp paprika
1 tsp cayenne pepper
1 tbsp nutritional yeast
1 tbsp fresh lime juice
Salt (or black salt)
and black pepper

Loaded Breakfast Burritos

Inspired by Mexican burritos, this is the ultimate breakfast treat. The chickpeas add great texture and protein while soaking up all the seasonings. Combined with the cherry tomato salsa, guacamole and spinach, and sprinkled with lime juice and coriander, all wrapped up in a delicious toasted tortilla, they make a wonderfully sustaining burrito to start the day. Adding black salt gives an egg-like flavour to satisfy any nostalgic cravings.

'SERRANA,' JESUS ALEJANDRO 'EL NIÑO' (FEAT. ARIEL BETANCOURT) –

First make the chickpea scramble. Gently warm the olive oil in a large saucepan, add the onion and red pepper and sauté over a medium heat for 6–7 minutes until lightly browned. Meanwhile, pulse the chickpeas in a blender or food processor until broken down slightly but not puréed. Alternatively, mash the chickpeas with a fork or potato masher.

Add the garlic, spices and nutritional yeast to the pan and stir in. Once the garlic has cooked down slightly, add the chickpeas, mix well to coat in the spices and cook for 5 minutes.

Remove from the heat, add ½ teaspoon of the black salt and the lime juice and mix together.

Lay out the tortillas and fill each with some of the spinach, guacamole, tomato salsa and chickpea scramble. Squeeze over one of the lime wedges and add a sprinkling of coriander, then season to taste with salt and pepper. Fold each filled tortilla into a burrito by folding in two opposite sides, then folding up the bottom part of the tortilla and rolling up to enclose the filling. Any leftover filling can be kept in the fridge for the next day.

Warm a dry non-stick frying pan over a medium heat. Place one burrito in the pan and cook for 3 minutes until the burrito is browned and toasted, then turn over and cook for another 3–5 minutes until toasted on the other side. Remove from the pan, then repeat with the remaining burritos and serve once all four have been toasted.

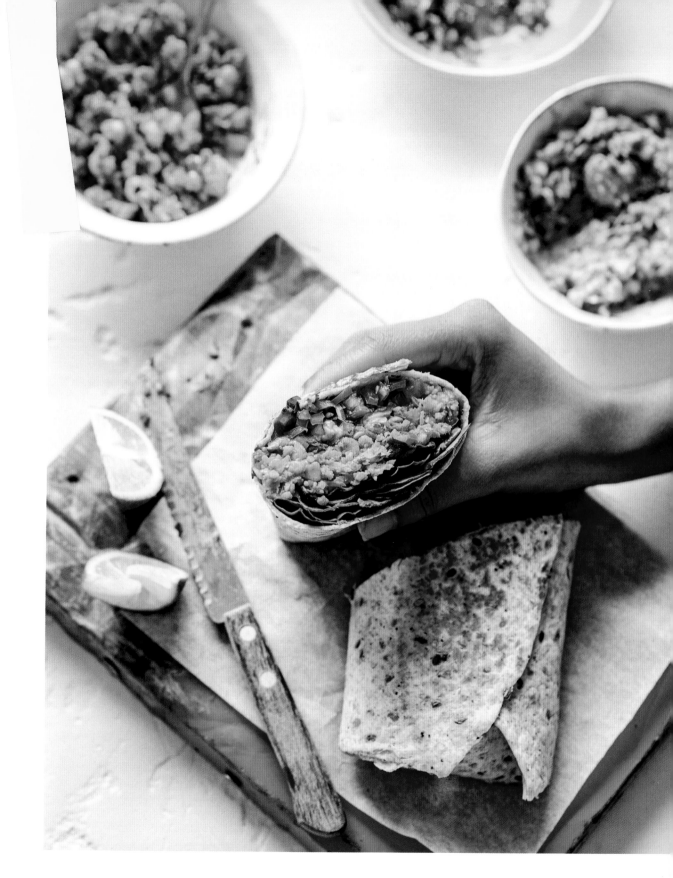

Serves 4

4 large tomatoes

2 avocados

8 slices of seeded wholemeal sourdough bread

8 tbsp vegan mayonnaise (to make your own, see pages 189 or 190)

8 leaves of butterhead lettuce

For the smoky aubergine

2 aubergines

1 tsp sweet smoked paprika

1 tsp garlic granules

1 tbsp liquid smoke (or soy sauce or coconut aminos)

1 tbsp soy sauce (or coconut aminos)

1 tsp vegan Worcestershire sauce

2 tbsp maple syrup

2 tbsp olive oil, plus extra for greasing

Salt and black pepper

Banging A(ubergine) LT Toasted Sandwiches

Fresh, crunchy and incredibly tasty, this has to be one of my favourite toasted vegan sandwiches. The sweet, smoky and slightly crispy aubergines pack so much flavour, offset by the juicy tomatoes, sliced avocado, lettuce and creamy mayo. Perfect for brunch or a light lunch. I used to be obsessed with a good BLT on occasion before going vegan and when I made this version with crispy aubergine I was blown away by how delicious it is!

Preheat the oven to 180°C fan, then line a baking sheet with baking paper or grease with olive oil.

Slice each aubergine in half lengthways, then slice each half in half again, giving you four long pieces of aubergine. Finely slice the aubergine pieces lengthways into strips 2–3mm thick.

Mix together all the other ingredients for the smoky aubergine in a bowl and season with salt and pepper. Brush the aubergine slices with the marinade, or dip them into the bowl, wiping off any excess, then spread on the prepared baking sheet in a single layer and cook in the oven for 15 minutes. Remove the baking sheet from the oven, brush both sides of the aubergine slices with an extra layer of marinade and return to the oven to cook for another 15 minutes.

Cook the aubergine slices for longer if you want them super-crispy, but keep an eye on them to ensure the maple syrup does not begin to burn. Once cooked, allow them to cool for a few minutes – the texture gets a little more chewy and crispy once cooled.

Meanwhile, slice the tomatoes and avocados and toast the bread. Spread four slices of toast with mayonnaise and divide between plates. To each piece of toast add a few sliced tomatoes and avocado and some of the smoky aubergine. Season to taste with salt and pepper, then top with two lettuce leaves and sandwich together with another slice of toast.

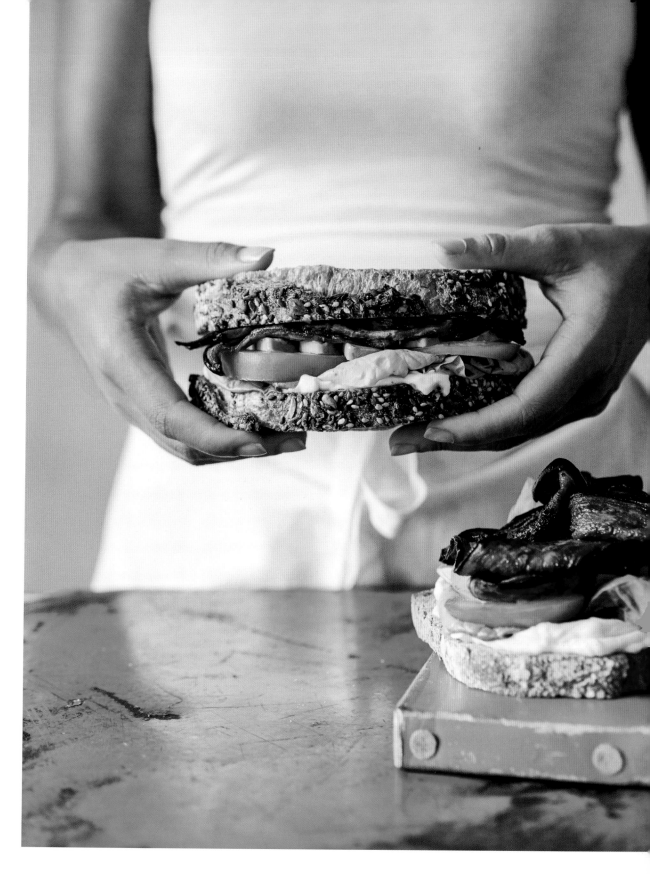

2

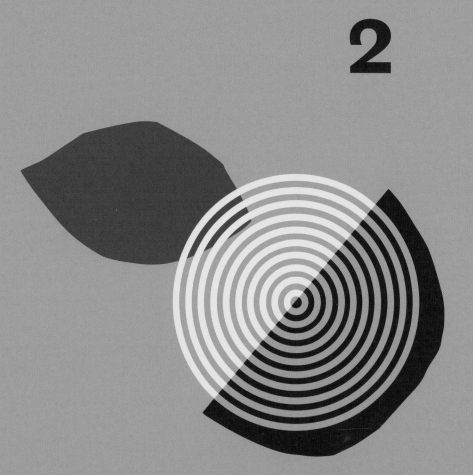

LUNCH AND LIGHT BITES

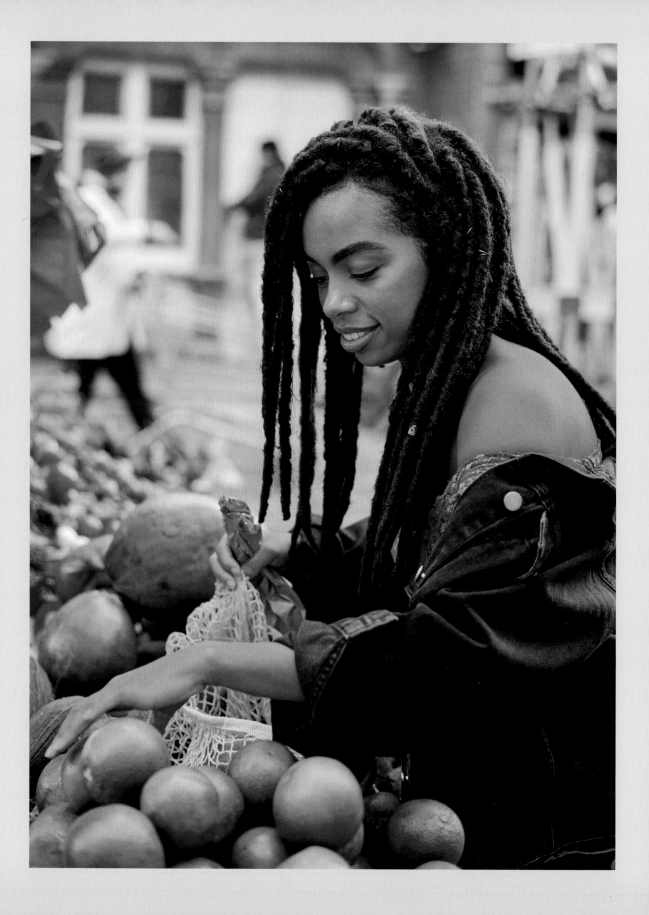

Lunch and Light Bites

Whether you want a wholesome, hearty filling lunch
or just a quick snack I've got lots of options for you.

Toasties are one of my favourite things to make for
a simple lunch, and wraps filled with fresh crunchy
vegetables and salads that you can make ahead
and then take on the go. The Corn Fritters with Tomato
and Avocado Salsa on page 68 are so flavourful and
another really easy way to get in some extra veggies!

If you've got guests coming over I highly recommend
the Chive Tofu Spread with Griddled Garlic Aubergines
on page 53 – it's so tasty and a great appetiser if you
want to give people something to munch on while
you finish the main dish.

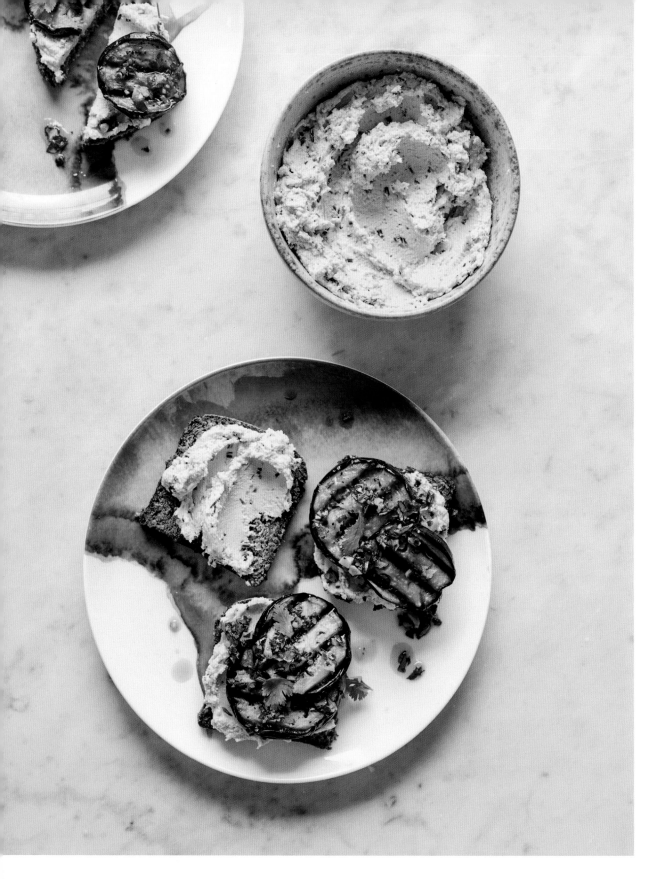

Lunch and Light Bites

Serves 4

1 tbsp olive oil
2 aubergines, each sliced
    into rounds 2cm thick
1 quantity of Chive Tofu
    Spread (see page 178)
8 slices of sprouted-
    grain bread
Salt and black pepper

**For the garlic-
chilli vinaigrette**
4 garlic cloves,
    finely chopped
1 tbsp olive oil
1 tbsp balsamic vinegar
2 tbsp extra-virgin olive oil
1 tsp maple syrup
1 tbsp fresh lemon juice
1 tsp chilli flakes

Handful of parsley,
    roughly chopped,
    plus extra to serve
Handful of coriander,
    roughly chopped,
    plus extra to serve

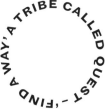

'FIND A WAY' A TRIBE CALLED QUEST –

Chive Tofu Spread with Griddled Garlic Aubergines

These super-tasty slices make the perfect flavoursome snack, as well as being great for serving as appetisers for a meal with friends. Sprouted-grain bread, such as Ezekiel, is made using a variety of whole grains and legumes that have begun to sprout, which makes it tasty and rich in healthy fibres and nutrients and is why I like to buy it from time to time as an alternative to regular bread. You can, however, enjoy the creamy tofu and grilled aubergines on any bread you like – seeded sourdough or rye bread both work well.

Heat up a griddle pan (or a heavy-based frying pan) and add the olive oil. Place the aubergines in the pan, season with salt and pepper and cook over a medium heat for 2–3 minutes until griddle lines appear, then turn over and continue to cook for another 2 minutes until tender.

In a separate pan, sauté the garlic for the vinaigrette in a tablespoon of olive oil over a medium heat for 3–4 minutes until softened.

Place the cooked garlic in a bowl, then pour in the balsamic vinegar, extra-virgin olive oil, maple syrup and lemon juice, add the chilli flakes and fresh herbs and mix well.

Toss the aubergines in the vinaigrette, reserving some for drizzling at the end.

Spread a generous amount of the chive tofu spread on each slice of bread and top with the dressed aubergines. Grind over some pepper and then sprinkle with the reserved vinaigrette and the extra parsley and coriander.

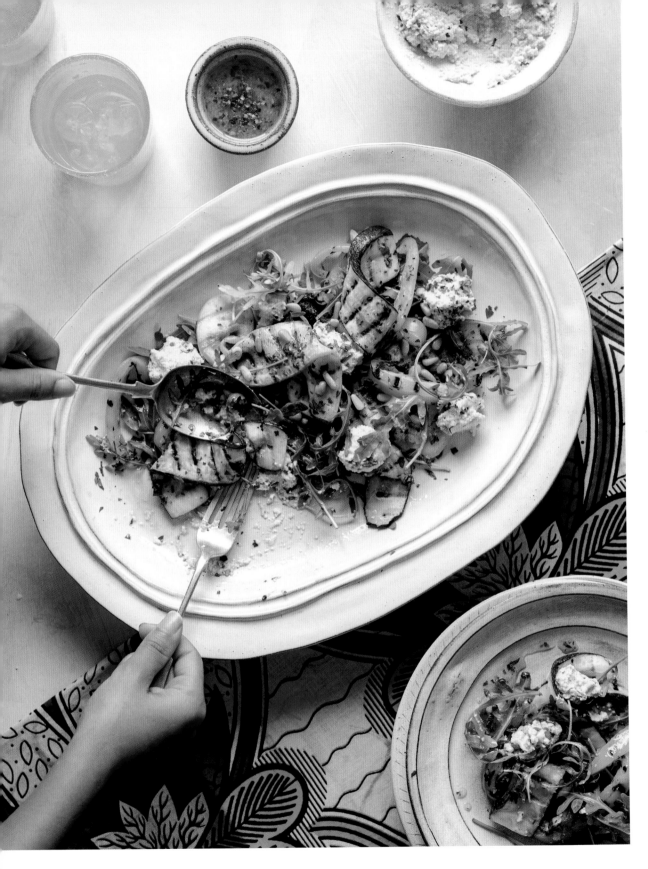

Lunch and Light Bites

Serves 4

2 large courgettes, cut lengthways into slices 3mm thick

1 yellow pepper, halved, deseeded and cut lengthways into thin strips

6 tbsp Basil Cashew Spread (see page 179)

For the dressing

2 tbsp extra-virgin olive oil

1 garlic clove, finely chopped

1 tsp chilli flakes

Small handful of fresh parsley, finely chopped

Small handful of fresh mint leaves, finely chopped

Juice of 1 lemon

Salt and black pepper

To serve

Handful of rocket leaves

Handful of pine nuts

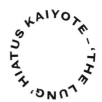

KAIYOTE – 'THE LUNG', HIATUS

Griddled Courgette and Pepper Salad with Rocket and Pine Nuts

In a large bowl, mix together all the ingredients for the dressing and season to taste with salt and pepper.

Heat a griddle pan (or a heavy-based frying pan) over a medium–high heat. Add the courgettes and peppers in a single layer (you might need to griddle them in batches) and cook for about 4 minutes on each side until lightly charred and just beginning to soften.

Add the griddled courgettes and peppers to the bowl with the dressing and toss together.

Spread the rocket leaves out in a large serving dish, then add the dressed courgettes and peppers, followed by the cashew spread (added as separate spoonfuls), the pine nuts and salt and pepper to taste.

Griddled courgettes and sweet yellow peppers in a super-tasty herb, lemon and garlic dressing, accompanied by peppery rocket and spoonfuls of creamy basil cashew spread topped with pine nuts. You can enjoy this is as a fresh light salad, or use it to fill a wrap or sandwich.

8 slices of sourdough bread

2 avocados

Handful of alfalfa sprouts

Juice of 1 lime

Handful of fresh coriander,
roughly chopped

For the chickpeas

1 tbsp olive oil

2 × 400g tins of chickpeas,
drained and rinsed

1 tbsp sweet smoked paprika

1 tsp garlic granules

½–1 tsp cayenne pepper
(to taste)

Juice and grated zest of
1 lime

Salt and black pepper

Avocado Toast with Crispy Chickpeas

Spice up your regular avocado on toast with these quick-and-easy addictive little crispy chickpeas!

First cook the chickpeas. Heat the olive oil in a pan, then add the chickpeas and sauté over a medium heat, stirring frequently, for 2–3 minutes. Add the smoked paprika, garlic granules, cayenne pepper, season with a little salt and continue to sauté for another 3–4 minutes until the chickpeas are golden brown and crispy. Remove the pan from the heat and stir in the lime juice and zest.

Meanwhile, toast the bread and divide between plates. Slice each avocado in half and remove the stone. Using a fork, lightly mash the avocado, then scoop out the flesh with a spoon and spread it on the toasted bread, seasoning to taste with salt and pepper.

Add some of the crispy chickpeas to each piece of avocado-covered toast, then sprinkle with alfalfa sprouts, lime juice and chopped coriander.

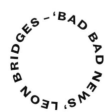

BRIDGES – 'BAD BAD NEWS', LEON

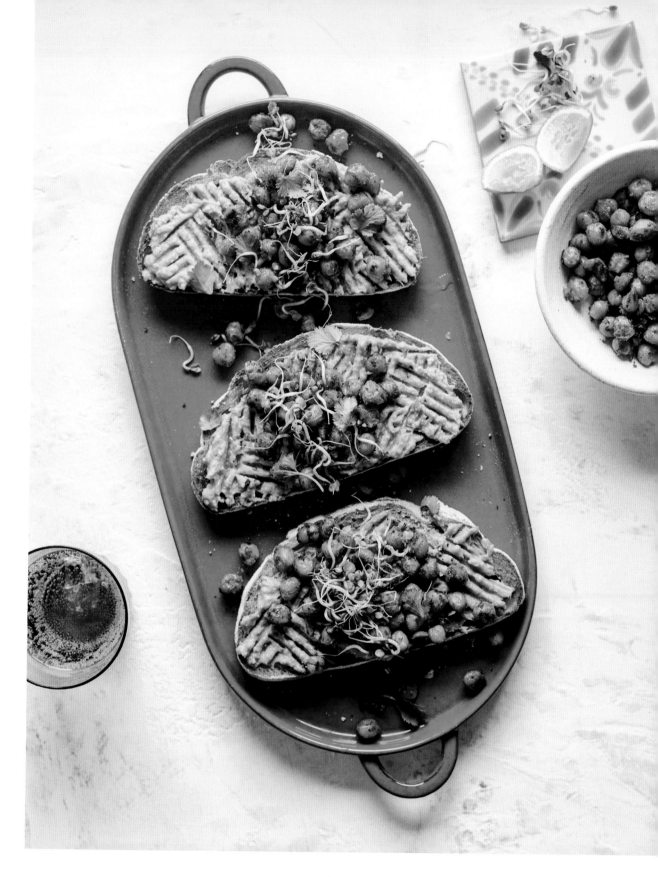

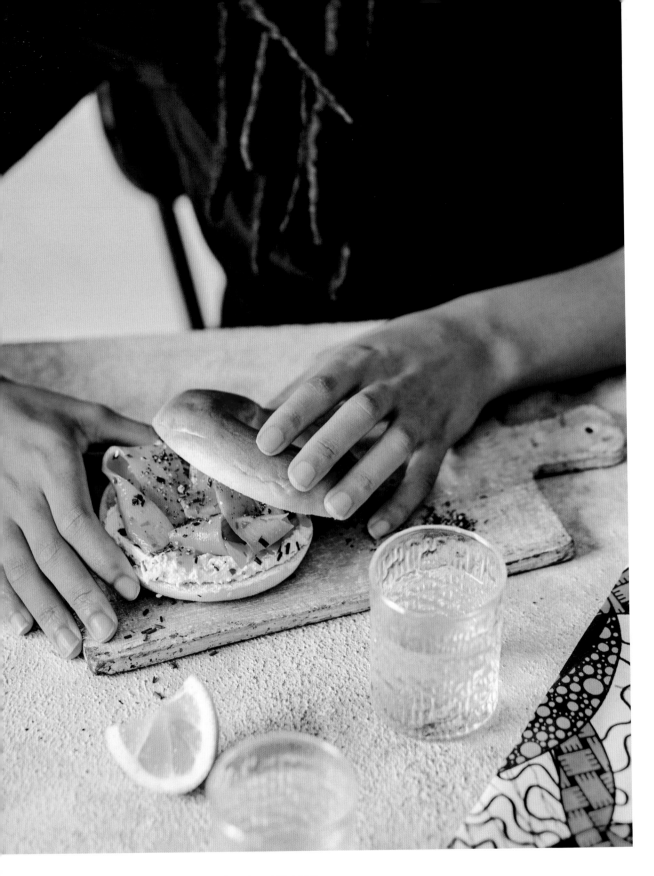

Lunch and Light Bites

Serves 4

1 quantity of Chive Tofu
   Spread (see page 178)
4 bagels, halved
1 tbsp finely snipped chives
1 lemon, cut into 4 wedges
Black pepper

For the smoked carrot
8 carrots
4 tbsp extra-virgin olive oil
2 tsp liquid smoke (or soy
   sauce or coconut aminos)
1 tbsp fresh lemon juice
1 tbsp soy sauce
   (or coconut aminos)
1 tbsp nori flakes
Salt

Smoked Carrot and Chive Tofu Bagels

My favourite kind of bagel. After becoming a vegan, I wanted to find a way to recreate the concept of smoked salmon and cream cheese. These marinated carrot slices do an amazing job of reproducing the smooth, fishy texture and flavour of smoked salmon, while the spread is creamy and thick, making this bagel a delicious alternative to the non-vegan classic. For a soy-free option, substitute with the Basil Cashew Spread on page 179.

Preheat the oven to 180°C fan.

Scrub or peel the carrots and either grate them into long strips or slice into pieces 5mm thick. Place in an ovenproof dish and sprinkle with salt, then cover with a lid and bake in the oven for 25 minutes until tender. If the carrots are still a little firm, bake for a few minutes longer. Remove from the oven and set aside to cool.

Place the olive oil, liquid smoke, lemon juice and soy sauce in a container with a lid, or a shallow bowl, add the nori and mix together well. Transfer the cooled carrots to the container/bowl, then massage the mixture into the carrots and seal the container with its lid, or cover the bowl with a plate, and store in the fridge for a minimum of 2 hours or preferably overnight for the best results.

Chill the chive tofu spread in the fridge for the last hour of the marinating time to help thicken the creamy tofu before serving.

Spread the chive tofu over the lower half of each bagel. Place the smoked carrot on top and sprinkle with some chives, squeeze over a lemon wedge and add a grind of black pepper before topping with the other bagel half.

Serves 4

4 large soft flour tortillas
1 quantity of Hummus
    (see page 177)
2 carrots, peeled and grated
½ cucumber, sliced
100g baby spinach
2 avocados, sliced
Juice of 1 lemon
Handful of fresh coriander,
    roughly chopped
Salt and black pepper

For the roasted vegetables

2 red peppers, thinly sliced
2 red onions, thinly sliced
1 tbsp olive oil
2 tbsp balsamic vinegar

Roasted Vegetable and Hummus Wraps

My go-to wrap for lunch! Crunchy fresh carrot and cucumber, home-made hummus, sweet roasted red onions and red peppers and creamy avocado with fresh lemon and coriander. All folded up in a soft flour tortilla to create this super-delicious wrap, bursting with different flavours and textures. Great for packed lunches too.

Preheat the oven to 180°C fan.

Place the red peppers and onions in an ovenproof pan or dish, add the olive oil and balsamic vinegar and mix in well so that the peppers and onions are well coated. Season with salt and pepper, cover with a lid and cook in the oven for 45 minutes or until tender. Remove from the oven and leave to cool down completely.

Lay out each tortilla and spread with a generous layer of hummus, then add some of the carrots, cucumber, spinach, avocado and roasted vegetables. Add a little lemon juice and salt and pepper to taste, sprinkle with the coriander and then make into a wrap by folding in two opposite sides, then folding up the bottom part of the tortilla and rolling up to enclose the filling.

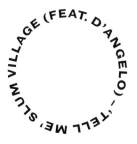
VILLAGE (FEAT. D'ANGELO) – 'TELL ME', SLUM

Serves 4

1 tbsp olive oil
8 slices of wholemeal bread
100g baby spinach
4 large tomatoes, sliced
4–6 slices of vegan hard
   cheese (a type that melts,
   such as vegan Cheddar)
50g vegan butter

For the basil pesto
120g basil leaves,
   roughly chopped
40g pine nuts
1 garlic clove,
   roughly chopped
1 tbsp nutritional yeast
1 tbsp fresh lemon juice
120ml extra-virgin olive oil
Salt and black pepper

Basil Pesto Tomato Toasties

Delicious toasties spread with fresh basil pesto and oozing with an irresistible mixture of sliced tomatoes, baby spinach and melted vegan cheese. The ultimate simple toasted sandwich. And yes, vegan cheese can melt and taste good! There are more and more vegan cheeses becoming available so look out for the ones that melt! When I don't have any vegan cheese sometimes I just sprinkle some nutritional yeast into the toasted sandwich instead, which is also super tasty.

Place all the pesto ingredients, except the extra-virgin olive oil, in a food processor and blend until roughly broken down – not a smooth paste. Pour the pesto into a bowl, mix in the extra-virgin olive oil and season to taste with salt and pepper.

Brush a griddle pan, frying pan or toastie maker with the tablespoon of olive oil to prevent the bread from sticking when toasted.

Spread a generous layer of pesto on one side of four slices of bread, then add the spinach and tomato slices and season with salt and pepper. Place an even layer of cheese on top and then close the sandwich with one of the remaining slices of bread.

Spread some butter on the outside of each sandwich and place, buttered side down, in the pan or toastie maker. If you are using a griddle pan or frying pan, I would recommend placing something heavy on top, such as a heavy saucepan, to weight the sandwich down as it cooks.

Cook over a medium heat for 3–4 minutes or until golden brown. Spread the top of the sandwich with more butter and then turn over to cook on the other side for another 2–3 minutes until golden brown and toasted all over. Slice in half to serve.

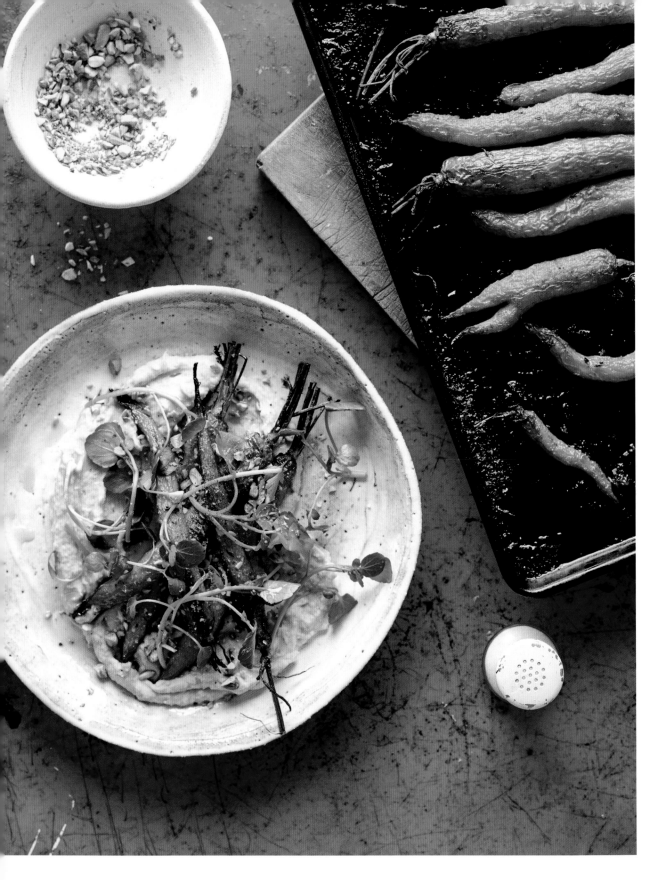

Lunch and Light Bites

400g carrots (unpeeled)
2 tbsp maple syrup
2 tbsp olive oil
1 tsp harissa paste
Grated zest of 1 lemon
Leaves from 2 thyme sprigs
Salt and black pepper

For the bean mash
1 tbsp olive oil,
    plus extra for drizzling
1 white onion, finely chopped
2 garlic cloves, finely chopped
2 × 400g tins of cannellini
    beans, drained and rinsed
Juice of ½ lemon

To serve
Large handful of watercress
Handful of pistachios,
    roughly chopped

Spiced Roasted Carrots with Garlic White Bean Mash

Who doesn't love a good roasted carrot? Here they are tossed in a sweet and spicy mixture of maple syrup and harissa before being roasted and then served dipped in a creamy white bean mash for a wonderfully tasty light lunch or snack!

Preheat the oven to 200°C fan.

Scrub the carrots and place in a roasting tin, add the maple syrup, olive oil, harissa paste, lemon zest and thyme and toss everything together so the carrots are well coated. Place in the oven to roast for 30–35 minutes, depending on the size of the carrots, until golden and caramelised and soft all the way through.

While the carrots are roasting, make the bean mash. Heat 1 tablespoon of the olive oil in a pan, add the onion and garlic and cook over a medium–low heat for about 5 minutes until softened. Stir in the cannellini beans to warm through and then remove from the heat and use a potato masher to mash together with the lemon juice and a drizzle of olive oil. Blend in a food processor for a really smooth mash.

Serve the roasted carrots and bean mash with the watercress and sprinkled with the pistachios.

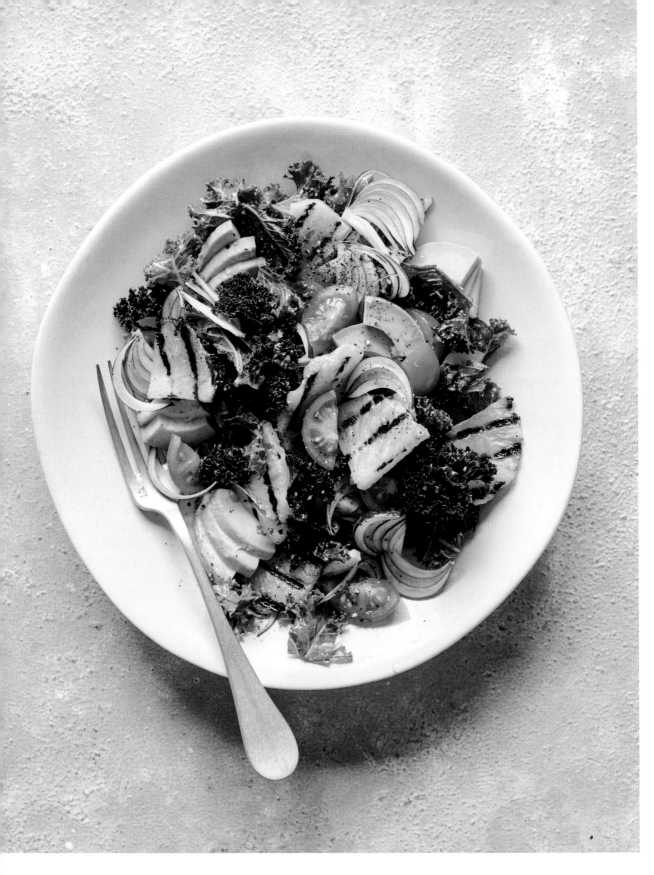

Lunch and Light Bites

Serves 4

200g kale, thick stalks
    removed and
    leaves chopped
1 tbsp fresh lemon juice
1 garlic cloves,
    finely chopped
1 tbsp extra-virgin olive oil

1 ripe pineapple
1 tbsp vegetable oil
1 red onion, finely sliced
300g cherry tomatoes,
    sliced in quarters
2 avocados, sliced
Salt and black pepper

Kale and Griddled Pineapple Salad

I definitely go through kale obsessions but if you are not sure about eating it raw, this fresh summery salad with a tropical touch is a great introduction to it. Massaging the kale with lemon, salt, pepper and a little olive oil not only brings out the flavour of the kale but also softens it and takes away potential bitterness. Combined with juicy, naturally sweet, griddled pineapples, avocado and cherry tomatoes, let the flavours take you away.

Place the kale in a bowl and combine with the lemon juice, garlic and olive oil. Sprinkle with salt and black pepper. With clean hands, massage the kale with your fingers for 2–3 minutes until the leaves start to soften, and then set aside while you prepare the rest of the dish.

Place the pineapple on a chopping board on its side and, using a large sharp knife, slice off the base of the fruit and the green top – cutting through the pineapple 1–2cm from the base of the leaves.

Stand the pineapple up and begin to carefully slice away the outer peel, cutting from top to bottom and following the contours of the pineapple. Lay the pineapple on its side and cut into 5cm-thick chunks.

Place a griddle pan (or a heavy-based frying pan) over a medium heat and add the vegetable oil. Add the pineapple chunks and cook for about 5 minutes on each side until heated through and lightly chargrilled.

To serve, place the griddled pineapple chunks in a serving bowl and combine with the softened kale, red onion, cherry tomatoes and avocados.

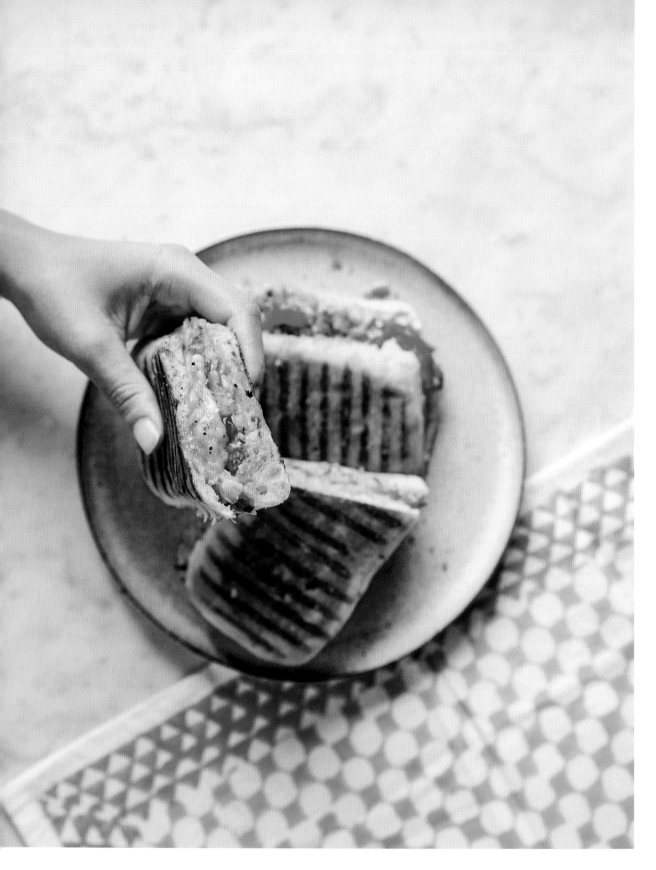

Lunch and Light Bites

Serves 4

1 tbsp olive oil
4 small ciabatta loaves
1 quantity of Chuna
    (see page 150)
4 large tomatoes, sliced

4–8 slices of vegan hard
    cheese (a type that melts,
    such as vegan Cheddar)
50g vegan butter
Salt and black pepper

Chuna Ciabatta Melts

I used to love making myself a tuna melt sandwich, so when I went vegan I was determined to devise a vegan version – enter my 'chuna': chickpea tuna (see page 150). I then combined it with vegan cheese (one that both tastes good and melts – major key) and sliced tomatoes in a classic toasted ciabatta. The result is a perfect, crunchy flavoursome sandwich to enjoy as a snack or for lunch. You can make this with regular bread too, if you like, and toast it in a toastie maker. Admittedly I used not to like vegan cheese, however, more and more good ones are being made. Believe it or not there are artisan vegan cheese shops in London where you can find some good-tasting vegan melty cheeses, but if you're looking for one you can get in most supermarkets, Violife has your back.

Brush a griddle pan, frying pan or toastie maker with the olive oil to prevent the toasted bread from sticking.

Slice each ciabatta in half horizontally and spread a generous amount of chuna on to the bottom half. Top with tomatoes and cheese, season with salt and pepper and then sandwich with the other half.

Spread some butter on the bottom of each filled ciabatta and place, buttered side down, in the pan or toastie maker. If you are using a griddle pan or frying pan, I would recommend placing something heavy on top, such as a heavy saucepan, to weight the sandwiches down as they cook (you might need to cook them in batches depending on the size of your pan).

Cook over a medium heat for 3–4 minutes or until golden brown. Spread the top of the loaf with more butter and then turn over to cook on the other side for another 2–3 minutes until golden brown and toasted all over. Slice in half to serve.

For the corn fritters

Kernels from 1 corn on
the cob
100g courgettes,
coarsely grated
150g peeled butternut
squash or carrots,
coarsely grated
100g polenta
1 tsp paprika
1 tsp ground cumin
2 spring onions, finely sliced

½ fresh red chilli, deseeded
and finely chopped
Small handful of fresh
coriander leaves,
roughly chopped
100ml oat milk (to make
your own, see page 238),
plus extra if needed
3 tbsp self-raising flour
2 flax eggs (see page 236)
Olive oil, for frying
Salt and black pepper

**For the tomato
and avocado salsa**

2 ripe tomatoes,
roughly chopped
1 avocado, chopped
1 red onion, finely diced
Small handful of fresh
coriander leaves,
roughly chopped
Juice and grated zest of
1 lime
2 tbsp extra-virgin olive oil

Corn Fritters with Tomato and Avocado Salsa

Crispy corn fritters, packed with veg and polenta
and served with a juicy tomato and avocado salsa
– a perfect pairing!

Place all the ingredients for the fritters in a large bowl,
season with salt and pepper and mix with a wooden
spoon until everything is combined, adding a little
more milk if the mixture seems too thick.

Heat a little olive oil in a large, non-stick frying pan.
Add 2 tablespoons of the mixture per fritter and then
flatten slightly to about 1cm thick. Fry over a medium
heat for 2–3 minutes or until crispy and brown on the
bottom, then flip over and cook for another 2–3 minutes
until crisp and golden on the other side. Repeat with
the remaining mixture, cooking in batches and adding
more oil to the pan as needed. Keep the fritters warm
on a baking sheet in the oven on a low heat while
you finish making them.

Meanwhile, mix all the ingredients for the tomato
and avocado salsa in a bowl, season with salt and
pepper and serve with the fritters.

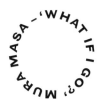

MURA MASA – 'WHAT IF I GO?'

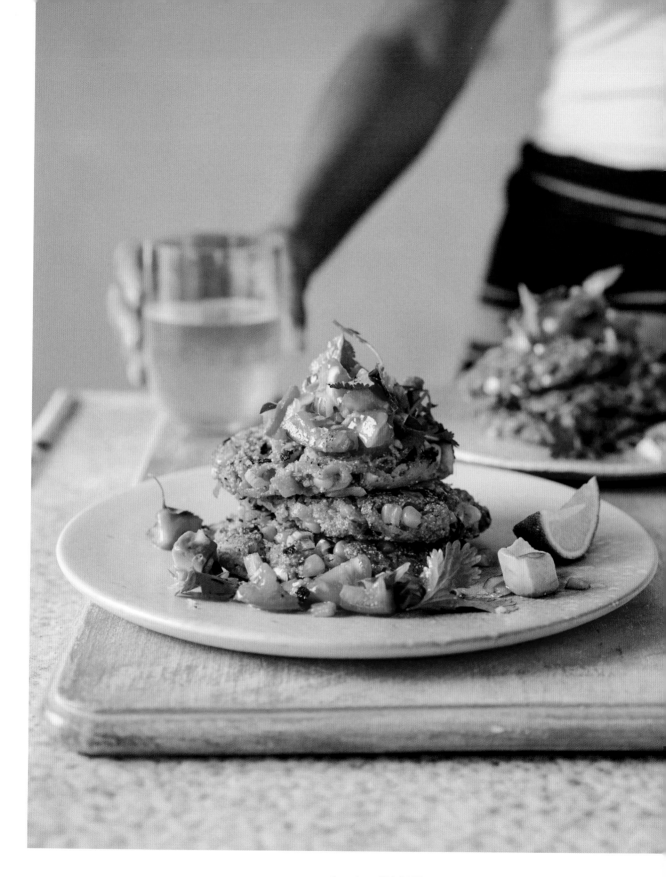

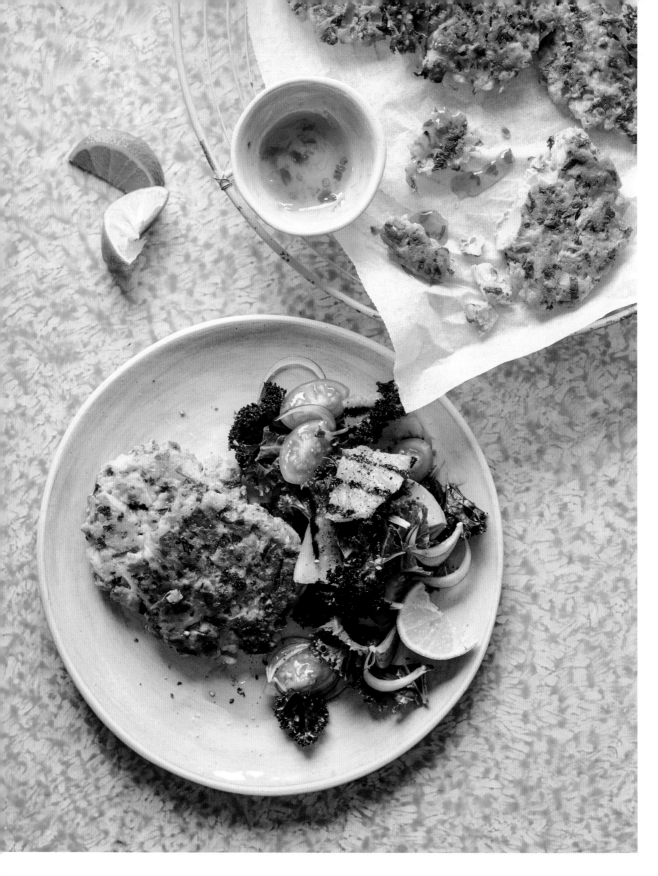

Lunch and Light Bites

Makes 8 fritters

1 × 400g tin of jackfruit,
　drained and rinsed
3 tbsp soy sauce
　(or coconut aminos)
2 tbsp nori flakes
2 tbsp fresh lemon juice
1 onion, finely chopped
2 spring onions,
　finely chopped
2 large tomatoes,
　finely chopped
2 mild red chillies, deseeded
　and finely chopped

3 garlic cloves,
　finely chopped
1 tsp dried thyme
Handful of coriander,
　finely chopped
Handful of parsley,
　finely chopped
1 tsp baking powder
190g chickpea flour
120ml water
Vegetable oil, for frying
Salt and black pepper

To serve
Sweet chilli sauce
1 quantity of Kale and
　Griddled Pineapple Salad
　(see page 65)

Caribbean Jackfruit Fritters

My grandma, who is from Saint Lucia, made the best fish fritters. My mum was completely addicted to them, so much so that as soon as she left college she and my dad planned to open a Caribbean restaurant in which my grandma would do the cooking. It didn't come to fruition in the end, though my grandma's cooking skills were unmatched. This is my take on her fish fritters but without the fish. Keeping my mum in mind, who is wheat intolerant, it also uses chickpea flour, which I believe really enhances the taste. I just love these little fritters. They're packed with flavour and full of nostalgia for me too, as they're so evocative of my grandma's. Perfect as a snack on their own or served with a salad.

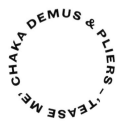

Using clean hands or a fork, break the jackfruit into small pieces, removing any tough stems, and then place in a bowl with the soy sauce, nori flakes and 1 tablespoon of the lemon juice. Mix well to combine, then cover the bowl with a plate and set aside.

Combine the onion and spring onions in a large bowl with the tomatoes, chillies, garlic, thyme and remaining lemon juice and then add the jackfruit mixture. Add the coriander and parsley and mix well.

Sift the baking powder and chickpea flour into a separate bowl, add the water, mix and season with salt and pepper before combining this with the jackfruit and onion mixture. The mixture should be slightly sloppy, so add a little more water if needed. Divide the mixture into eight and shape with your hands into small flat cakes, each about 1cm thick.

Pour a little vegetable oil into a large frying pan set over a medium heat.

Carefully place as many cakes as will fit in a single layer in the pan without touching. Cook for about 5 minutes, until golden brown on the bottom, then turn over and cook for another 5 minutes until crisp and cooked all the way through. Fry the fritters in batches, using a little more oil as needed and keeping them warm on a baking sheet in the oven on a low heat. (Make sure that the oven isn't too hot, or the fritters will dry out.) Serve with sweet chilli sauce and the kale and griddled pineapple salad.

Makes 8–10 falafels

400g sweet potatoes
   (unpeeled)
280g dried chickpeas,
   soaked overnight
2 tsp ground cumin
1 tsp ground coriander
4 garlic cloves,
   roughly chopped
1 tbsp harissa paste
1 tbsp fresh lemon juice

Handful of fresh parsley,
   roughly chopped
Handful of fresh coriander,
   roughly chopped
40–80g chickpea flour
50g fresh wholemeal
   breadcrumbs
Vegetable oil, for deep-frying
Salt and black pepper

Chickpea Sweet Potato Falafels

Who doesn't love a good falafel? This recipe combines chickpeas with sweet potato for extra flavour and texture. Mixed with cumin, coriander and fresh herbs, and a spoonful of harissa paste for a little heat, these falafels are gorgeous and can be eaten hot or cold. I love them inside pitta with a layer of hummus and salad, and they are very handy to keep in the fridge – just dip in a little hummus and you have a complete snack! This recipe works best with dried chickpeas.

Preheat the oven to 180°C fan. Prick the sweet potatoes with a fork, place on a baking tray and bake in the oven for about 45 minutes or until tender. Let the sweet potatoes cool, then slice in half, scoop out the insides and place these in a food processor.

Drain and rinse the soaked chickpeas, then add them to the food processor, along with all the remaining ingredients except for the flour and breadcrumbs. Season with salt and pepper and pulse until well mixed but still quite coarse. Check the seasoning and add more salt and pepper if needed.

Tip in half the chickpea flour and pulse again. Pinch off some of the mixture and, using your hands, roll into a small ball to test the consistency. If it is too sticky and wet, add as much of the remaining chickpea flour as needed. Place the falafel mixture in a bowl, cover with a plate and place in the fridge to firm up for 1–2 hours.

Pour enough of the oil into a large, heavy-based saucepan to a depth of 3–5cm and heat until it reaches 180°C on a thermometer. Or drop in a cube of bread and, if it cooks in 30–40 seconds, the oil should be hot enough. Roll the falafel mixture into 8–10 balls about 4cm wide, then roll them in the breadcrumbs to coat.

Carefully lower the falafels into the hot oil with a slotted spoon and fry for 5–6 minutes, turning, until browned all over. (You may need to fry them in batches – they should form a single layer in the pan without touching each other.) Remove from the oil and drain on kitchen paper to soak up any excess oil. Serve hot or cold.

Makes 4 full tortillas

Vegetable oil, for frying
8 large soft flour tortillas
16 slices of vegan hard
    cheese (a type that melts,
    such as vegan Cheddar)
1 quantity of Mango
    Avocado Salsa
    (see page 181), to serve

For the coriander pesto
100g fresh coriander,
    roughly chopped
2 garlic cloves,
    roughly chopped
4 spring onions,
    roughly chopped
1 fresh green chilli, deseeded
    and roughly chopped
1 tsp ground coriander
½ tsp ground cumin
1 tbsp nutritional yeast
120ml extra-virgin olive oil
Salt and black pepper

Griddled Cheesy Coriander Pesto Tortillas

Growing up, whenever summertime hit London, my mum would get out the barbecue and make these for me because she knew how much I loved them. Summer was officially here when I'd smell them cooking. Coriander pesto with a few green chillies for spice, and vegan cheese (one that both tastes good and melts) are used here to fill the tortillas, which are then toasted, melting the cheese and leaving the outside nice and crispy. Slice them up just before serving and spoon over a generous amount of fresh mango avocado salsa to offset the chilli pepper in the pesto with a touch of sweetness – so, so scrumptious!

Place all the pesto ingredients, except the olive oil, in a food processor and blend until roughly broken down – not a smooth paste. Pour the pesto into a bowl, mix in the olive oil and season to taste with salt and pepper.

Preheat a griddle pan (or a heavy-based frying pan) and brush with vegetable oil to prevent the tortillas from sticking while toasting.

Spread one tortilla with a generous portion of coriander pesto, then cover with a layer of cheese slices and lightly press a second tortilla on top to sandwich together. Repeat with the remaining tortillas, keeping them flat rather than folding them.

Place a filled tortilla in the pan and cook over a medium heat for about 2 minutes or until lightly charred and the cheese has melted slightly. Carefully flip over and cook for another 2 minutes on the other side until lightly charred all over.

Cut the filled tortillas into quarters and serve with the mango avocado salsa.

Serves 4

1 tbsp vegetable oil
1 onion, finely sliced
1 red pepper, deseeded
    and finely sliced
1 yellow pepper, deseeded
    and finely sliced
2 spring onions, sliced
Leaves from 2 thyme sprigs
4 garlic cloves,
    finely chopped
1 fresh red chilli, deseeded
    and finely chopped

2 × 410g tins of hearts
    of palm, drained and
    finely sliced
2 tbsp soy sauce
    (or coconut aminos)
1 tbsp fresh lemon juice
3 tbsp nori flakes
2 medium tomatoes,
    roughly chopped
1 × 540g tin of ackee, drained
Salt and black pepper

To serve
Handful of parsley,
    finely chopped
2 avocados, sliced (optional)
1 lime, cut into 4 wedges
1 quantity of Caribbean
    Dumplings (see page 149)

Ackee 'Saltfish' with Caribbean Dumplings

A vegan take on a classic Caribbean breakfast. Instead of the original salty fish, this recipe uses hearts of palm, which have a very subtle, savoury flavour and hold their shape well, soaking up all the traditional seasonings in the dish. For the sea-like flavours, I use nori flakes combined with ackee, the national fruit of Jamaica, which also has a very subtle taste. Be careful not to over-mix the ackee as it breaks apart quite easily. Serve with Caribbean Dumplings (Johnny cakes, see page 149) and I always add a few slices of avocado too.

Heat the vegetable oil in a large frying pan, add the onions and sauté over a low heat for 5 minutes, then add the red and yellow peppers, spring onions, thyme, garlic and chilli and cook for 7–8 minutes until tender.

Tip in the palm hearts, add the soy sauce, lemon juice and nori flakes and mix to combine. Mix in the tomatoes and then gently stir in the ackee, taking care not to let it break up. Season to taste with salt and pepper and then leave to heat through for 4–5 minutes before removing from the heat.

Sprinkle with the parsley and serve with the avocado (if using), the lime wedges for squeezing over and the sweet fried dumplings.

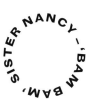

SISTER NANCY – 'BAM BAM'

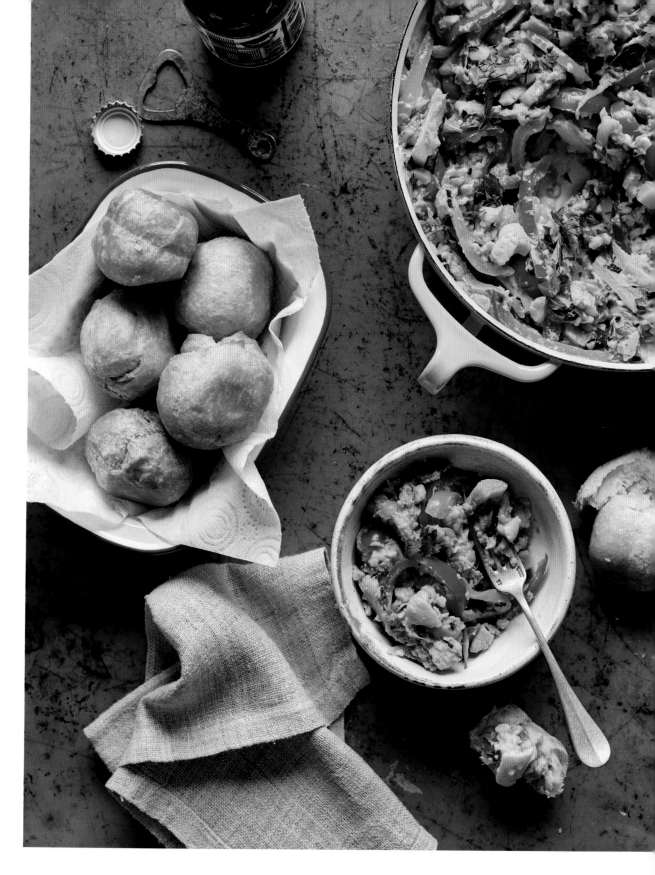

Serves 4

4 large potatoes (such as
    Maris Piper, King Edward
    or Estima), unpeeled
4 tbsp vegan butter
4 tbsp nutritional yeast
Salt and black pepper

For the salad
Handful of salad leaves,
    roughly chopped
2 avocados, sliced
Handful of cherry tomatoes,
    quartered
100g alfalfa sprouts

For the vinaigrette
200ml extra-virgin olive oil
60ml fresh lemon juice or
    balsamic vinegar
1 garlic clove, grated
½ tsp Dijon mustard
1 tsp maple syrup

To serve
1 quantity of Chuna
    (see page 150)
1 lemon, cut into 4 wedges

Chuna Jacket Potatoes with Salad

Jacket potatoes with crisp, crunchy skins and fluffy middles have always been a love of mine. I often turned to them as a student for delicious comfort and ease. These are topped with my chickpea-based 'chuna' mayo, which tastes so much like the original tuna version – but better! A quick and simple yet filling meal.

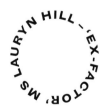

Preheat the oven to 220°C fan.

Wash the potatoes well and prick here and there with a fork, then place on a baking tray, sprinkle with a pinch of salt then bake on the middle shelf of the oven for about 1 hour or until the potatoes just give as you squeeze them and their skins are crisp.

Remove from oven and cut a cross on the top of each potato, then gently squeeze the sides until it pops open. Place a tablespoon of butter inside each potato, sprinkle over a tablespoon of the nutritional yeast and season with salt and pepper.

Mix together the salad ingredients in a bowl. Combine the ingredients for the vinaigrette in another bowl and season to taste with salt and vinegar. Drizzle the dressing over the salad and toss together well.

Serve each baked potato with a spoonful of chuna, a wedge of lemon and with some of the salad alongside.

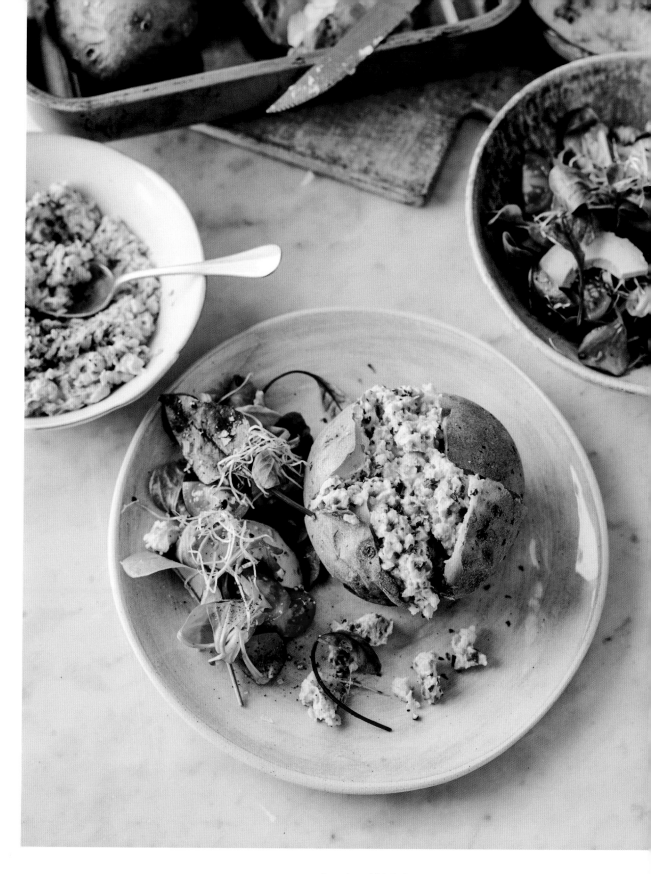

3

DINNER

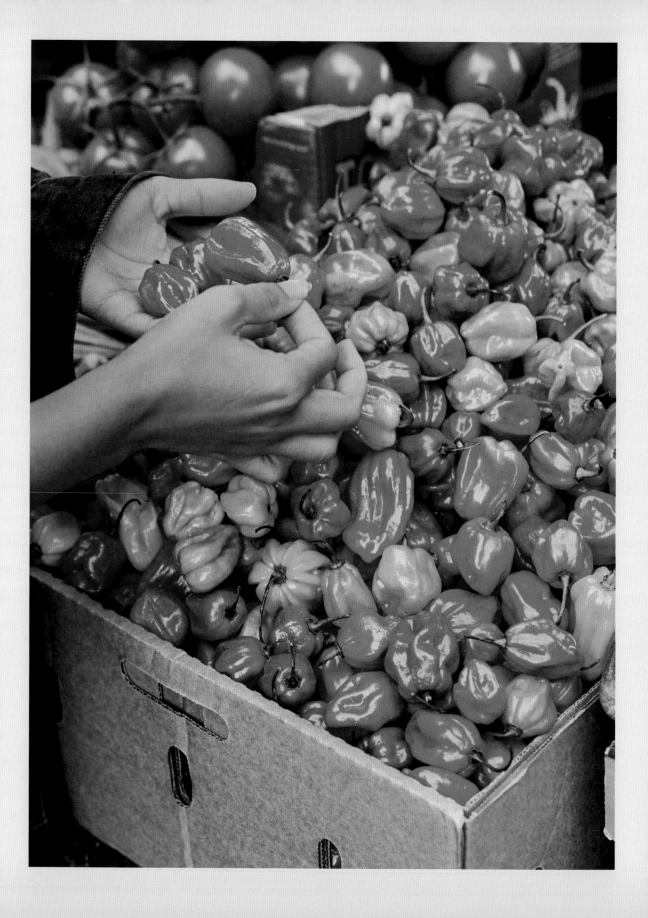

Dinner

Dinner is my favourite meal – the big finale to put my taste buds in a good mood after a long day – and I love a good, hearty comforting dish.

The rich stews, fragrant curries and pasta dishes in this chapter definitely have you covered. I usually make one of them in a big batch at the start of the week and then eat them over the next few days when I don't have much time to prep and cook.

You'll also find some delicious fresh salads with a variety of vegetables, dressings and herbs to make them super-tasty. You'll notice I like to use a lot of different grains in my salads – for flavour and to keep them more filling, as much as for their nutritional value.

There are a few big recipes that take a little longer to prepare than your quick everyday essentials – recipes such as the Tabbouleh Salad Feast and Jerk Mushroom and Caramelised Onion Feast (see pages 91 and 138) – but they're seriously worth it and especially great for making when you have guests and want to share a big, delicious plant-based meal.

Serves 4

1 tbsp olive oil
1 large onion, finely chopped
1 leek, finely chopped
1 garlic clove, finely chopped
Leaves from 2 thyme sprigs
2 celery sticks,
    finely chopped and saving
    the leaves to garnish
1 courgette, diced
    into 2cm chunks

Handful of fresh parsley,
    stalks and leaves
    separated and
    roughly chopped
1 bay leaf
750ml vegetable stock
2 × 400g tins of butter beans,
    drained and rinsed
300g mixed greens (such
    as spinach, cavolo nero,
    Swiss chard, watercress
    or kale), roughly chopped
Juice of ½ lemon

For the parsnip crisps
1 large parsnip
1 tbsp olive oil
Salt and black pepper

All-greens Chunky Butter Bean Soup with Parsnip Crisps

This super-tasty broth-like soup is perfect on colder days or for when you're feeling a little under the weather and in need of a warming and healthy pick-me-up. Use a combination of whatever you have in the fridge for the greens – anything goes!

ERYKAH BADU – 'ON & ON'

Preheat the oven to 180°C fan.

First make the parsnip crisps. Peel the parsnip then use a vegetable peeler to shave the rest of it into long, thin strips. Add the parsnip strips to a large roasting tin, drizzle with the olive oil, season with salt and pepper and use your hands to mix everything together, so the parsnip strips are evenly coated. Spread the strips out into a single layer and then place in the oven to roast for 20 minutes or until crispy and golden.

Meanwhile, prepare the soup. Place the olive oil in a large saucepan, add the onion, leek, garlic, thyme and celery and fry over a medium heat for 5 minutes until softened. Add the courgette, parsley stalks and bay leaf and sauté for a further 3 minutes, then pour in the vegetable stock and butter beans. Season with salt and pepper and bring to the boil, then reduce the heat to simmer for another 10 minutes.

Tip in the mixed greens and cook for 2–3 minutes until wilted. Add the parsley leaves and lemon juice, then remove the bay leaf and taste for seasoning, adding more salt and pepper if needed.

Spoon into individual bowls and top with the parsnip crisps and reserved celery leaves.

Dinner

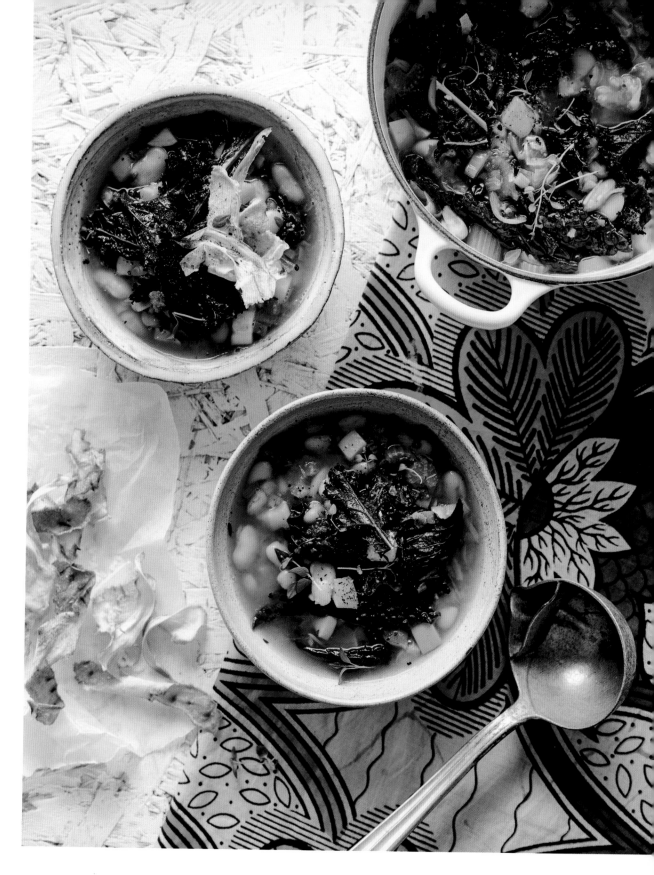

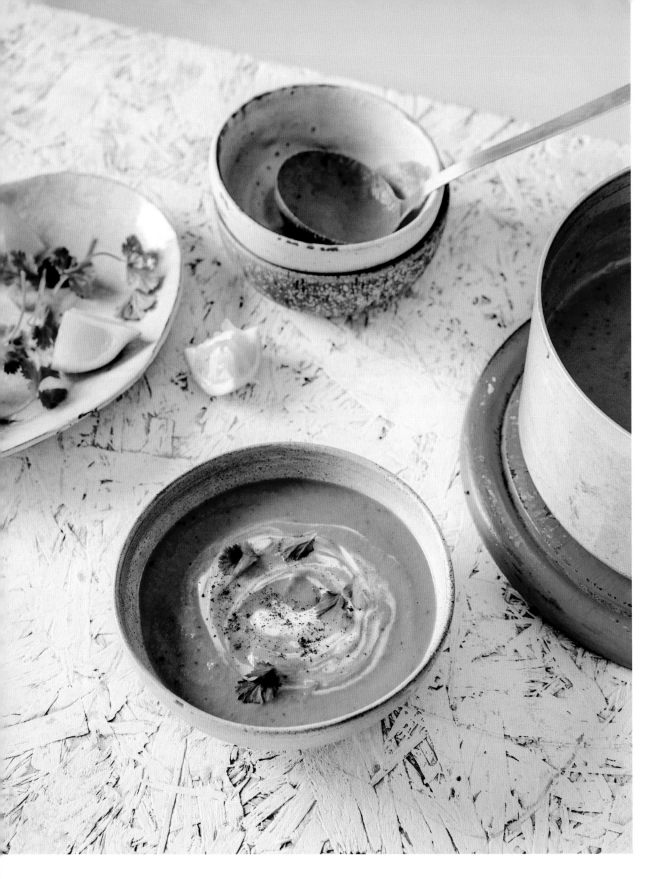

Dinner

Serves 4

1 tbsp coconut oil
2 onions, sliced
Thumb-sized piece
of fresh root ginger,
peeled and sliced
4 garlic cloves, sliced
2 tsp Madras curry powder
1 tsp ground turmeric
½ tsp cayenne pepper

1 tsp black mustard seeds
1 × 400g tin of chopped
tomatoes
200ml coconut milk
1 × 400g tin of chickpeas,
drained and rinsed
700g peeled butternut
squash, cut into chunks
Salt and black pepper

To serve

Handful of fresh coriander,
roughly chopped
1 tbsp fresh lemon juice
60g unsweetened vegan
coconut yoghurt

Curried Butternut Squash Soup

A thick creamy soup made with chickpeas, coconut milk, butternut squash and fragrant spices to warm you up. This nourishing soup is perfect in the autumn with a slice of fresh bread. You could also enjoy it as a curry by not blending it into a soup after cooking. Sometimes I eat this as a curry and then blend the leftovers into a soup for a variation.

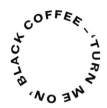

Melt the coconut oil in a saucepan, add the onions and mix to coat thoroughly in the oil. Sauté over a medium heat for 7–10 minutes, stirring occasionally, until the onions are softened and start to caramelise.

Add the ginger and garlic, reduce the heat a little and sauté for 3–4 minutes until the garlic is almost translucent and has absorbed the oil. Now add all the spices and stir in well. If the onions look close to burning, stir in 1–2 tablespoons of water and mix well, taking care not to burn the spices either.

Pour in the tinned tomatoes and coconut milk, add the chickpeas and butternut squash and season with salt and pepper. Mix well, cover with a lid and bring to the boil, then reduce the heat and cook for 20 minutes on a low simmer until the butternut squash is tender. Remove the lid and simmer over a low heat for another 10 minutes.

Remove from the heat and blend in a food processor, or using a hand blender, to the desired consistency.

To serve, divide between bowls and then sprinkle with the coriander and lemon juice, season with pepper and add a spoonful of the coconut yoghurt.

Serves 4

500g oyster mushrooms, roughly chopped
1 tbsp soy sauce (or coconut aminos)
2 tbsp vegan butter
2 large corn on the cob
Handful of fresh coriander, roughly chopped
2 limes, each cut into 4 wedges, to serve

For the chimichurri paste
2 spring onions, finely chopped
60g fresh coriander, finely chopped
40g fresh parsley, finely chopped
4 garlic cloves, finely chopped
1 fresh red chilli, deseeded and finely chopped
2 tbsp dried oregano

120ml extra-virgin olive oil
1 tbsp maple syrup
3 tbsp vegan red wine vinegar (or balsamic vinegar or fresh lemon juice)
Salt and black pepper

For the salad
2 avocados, sliced
4 handfuls of salad leaves
½ red onion, finely sliced
4 tomatoes, finely sliced

MURA MASA (FEAT. OCTAVIAN) – 'MOVE ME'

Chimichurri Mushroom and Sweetcorn Salad Bowl

Chimichurri is a classic South American herb paste made with chillies, fresh coriander and parsley and dried oregano and is so delicious. Here it adds bags of flavour to the slightly crispy roasted oyster mushrooms. Served with salad leaves, avocado and griddled sweetcorn kernels, they make a truly tasty salad bowl. Make sure you mix all the ingredients together thoroughly so that you get all the flavours in each mouthful! The chimichurri paste also works well on chargrilled or roasted vegetables.

Preheat the oven to 180°C fan.

First make the chimichurri paste. Use a pestle and mortar to roughly blend the spring onions, coriander, parsley, garlic, chilli and oregano. Season with salt and pepper, add the olive oil, maple syrup and red wine vinegar and mix well to combine. Alternatively, blitz all the ingredients together in a food processor. Taste and add more salt and pepper if needed.

Spread the mushrooms on a baking tray in a single layer and place in the oven to cook for 20 minutes, then remove from the oven and mix with 2 tablespoons of the chimichurri paste and the soy sauce. Spread out again on the baking tray and bake in the oven for another 15 minutes until browned and slightly crispy.

Meanwhile, melt the butter in a griddle pan (or a heavy-based frying pan) over a medium–high heat. Add the corn on the cob, season with salt and pepper and cook for about 7 minutes, turning frequently, until chargrilled all over. Transfer to a chopping board and allow to cool slightly, then, supporting each piece of corn at a 45-degree angle, run a sharp knife down each side from top to bottom to slice off the kernels.

Place all the salad ingredients in a serving bowl, then sprinkle with the coriander and drizzle with the remaining chimichurri sauce. Mix well and serve each portion with a couple of lime wedges.

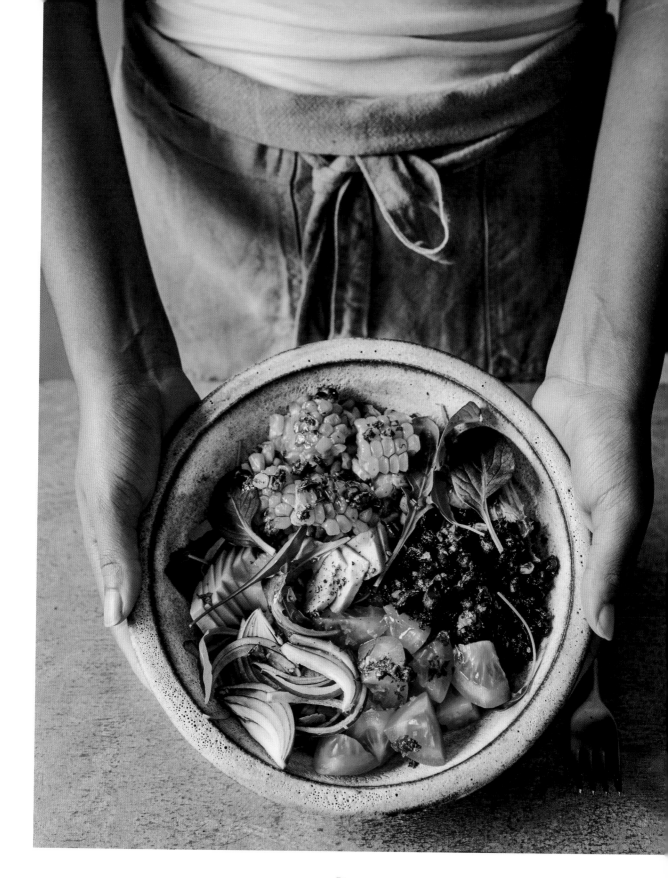

250g quinoa
2 limes, each cut into
    4 wedges
2 tbsp extra-virgin olive oil
1 tbsp vegetable oil
4 corn on the cob
2 avocados, sliced
600g cherry tomatoes,
    quartered

½ red onion, finely sliced
1 ripe mango,
    roughly chopped
Handful of fresh coriander,
    roughly chopped
2 fresh red chillies, deseeded
    and finely chopped
120g raw cashew nuts,
    roughly crushed
Salt and black pepper

Mango Quinoa Salad

A refreshing mixture of quinoa with tropical mangos, avocado, cherry tomatoes and grilled sweetcorn. Perfect in the summertime as a light, wholesome and tasty salad.

Rinse the quinoa well under the cold tap, then place in a saucepan with double the amount of water. Season with salt and bring to the boil, then reduce the heat, cover with a lid and simmer for 10–15 minutes, until the quinoa is tender and all the liquid has been absorbed. Fluff up with a fork, and transfer to a bowl to cool completely.

Once cool, squeeze in the juice from a wedge of lime, add the olive oil and season with salt and pepper. Leave to sit and marinate.

Meanwhile, preheat the grill to high, or place a griddle pan over a medium–high heat, and add the vegetable oil. Place the corn on the cob in the grill pan or griddle pan and cook, turning frequently, for 7–10 minutes until charred all over. Season with salt and pepper.

Transfer the corn on the cob to a chopping board and, with a sharp knife and supporting the corn at a 45-degree angle, cut downwards from the top to the bottom with a gentle sawing motion to remove the kernels, cutting to roughly two-thirds of the depth of the kernels.

Add the quinoa to a large serving plate or bowl, followed by the avocado, cherry tomatoes, red onion and mango, and then mix everything together. Sprinkle over the coriander, chillies and cashew nuts and squeeze over the juice of the lime wedges to serve.

Serves 4

2 × 400g tins of brown lentils,
  drained and rinsed
½ cucumber, finely sliced
1 red onion, finely chopped
1 red pepper, deseeded and
  finely chopped
4 large tbsp Basil Pesto
  (see page 61)
Juice of ½ lemon
Salt and black pepper

For the salad

Handful of salad leaves
300g cherry tomatoes,
  quartered
2 avocados, sliced
Handful of alfalfa sprouts
3 tbsp pumpkin seeds
2 tbsp extra-virgin olive oil
Juice of 1 lemon

To serve

1 quantity of Crispy New
  Potatoes (see page 163),
  to serve

Basil Pesto Lentils and Salad with Crispy New Potatoes

In a bowl, mix the lentils with the cucumber, red onion, red pepper and basil pesto. Add the lemon juice and season to taste with salt and pepper.

Place the salad leaves in a bowl with the tomatoes, avocados, alfalfa sprouts and pumpkin seeds, then dress with the olive oil and lemon juice, season to taste with salt and pepper and toss together well.

Serve the lentils with the salad and the crispy new potatoes.

This is one of my go-to meals in the summer – if you follow me on Instagram you've probably seen it on my feed! Mixing a pesto through lentils is a great way to add refreshing herby flavours to them and they are great matched with some crispy-on-the-outside, fluffy-on-the-inside new potatoes and a simple, crunchy salad.

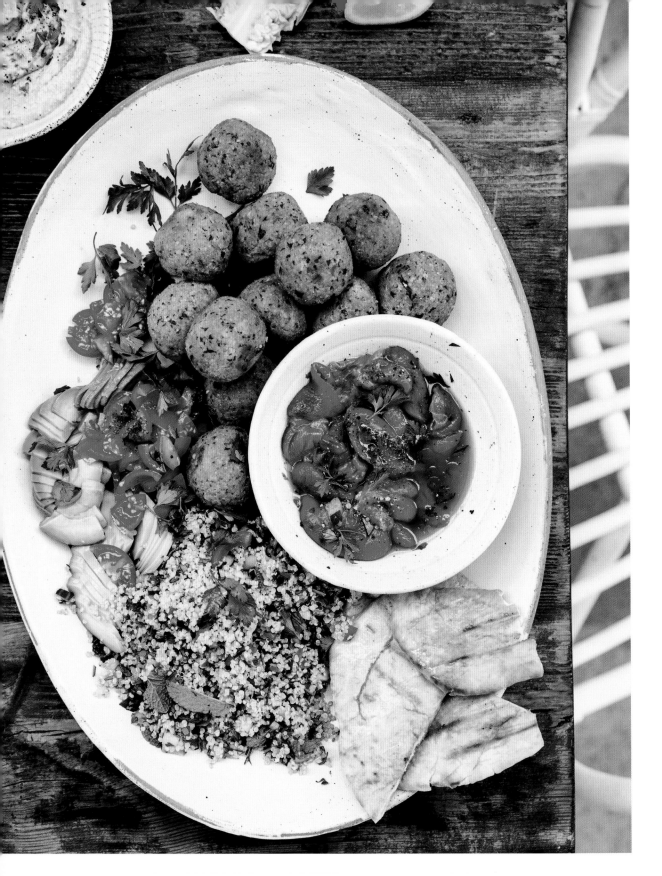

Serves 4

For the tabbouleh
100g fresh parsley,
    finely chopped
100g fresh coriander,
    finely chopped
10g fresh mint leaves,
    finely chopped
½ red onion, finely chopped
4 tomatoes, finely chopped
¼ cucumber, finely chopped
Juice of ½ lemon
2 tbsp extra-virgin olive oil
180g quinoa
Salt and black pepper

For the tahini dressing
120ml tahini
1 tbsp fresh lemon juice
1 tbsp extra-virgin olive oil
2 tbsp water
1 tsp maple syrup
Handful of fresh parsley,
    finely chopped

For the salad
Handful of salad leaves,
    roughly chopped
Handful of cherry tomatoes,
    quartered
2 avocados, sliced

To serve
1 quantity of Hummus
    (see page 177)
1 quantity of Roast Red
    Peppers (see page 154)
1 quantity of Chickpea
    Sweet Potato Falafels
    (see page 72)
1 lemon, cut into 4 wedges
Handful of fresh parsley,
    roughly chopped
4 pitta breads, toasted and
    sliced into quarters

Tabbouleh Salad Feast

Inspired by the classic Middle Eastern dish, this recipe uses quinoa marinated in a mixture of lemon juice and fresh, very finely chopped herbs, tomatoes and cucumbers. It is so simple and tasty, I just can't get enough of it! I love combining tabbouleh with hummus, falafels, roasted red peppers and warm pitta breads for a feast – especially good for serving to friends at a summer picnic.

In a large bowl, combine the fresh herbs, red onion, tomatoes and cucumber. Season with salt and pepper and add the lemon juice and olive oil. Mix well, cover with a plate and set aside to marinate while you prepare the quinoa.

Rinse the quinoa well under the cold tap, then place it in a saucepan with double the amount of water. Season with salt and bring to the boil, then reduce the heat, cover with a lid and simmer for 10–15 minutes, until the quinoa is tender and all the liquid has been absorbed. Fluff up the grains with a fork, and place in a bowl to cool completely.

Once cooled, add the quinoa to the bowl with the herb mixture, mix well and then taste, adding more salt and pepper if needed.

Mix all the ingredients for the tahini dressing in a bowl, seasoning to taste with salt and pepper. Combine all the salad ingredients in another bowl.

Transfer the tabbouleh to a serving dish and serve with the salad and separate bowls of hummus, red peppers, falafels, lemon wedges and chopped parsley. Serve the tahini dressing and toasted pitta bread alongside.

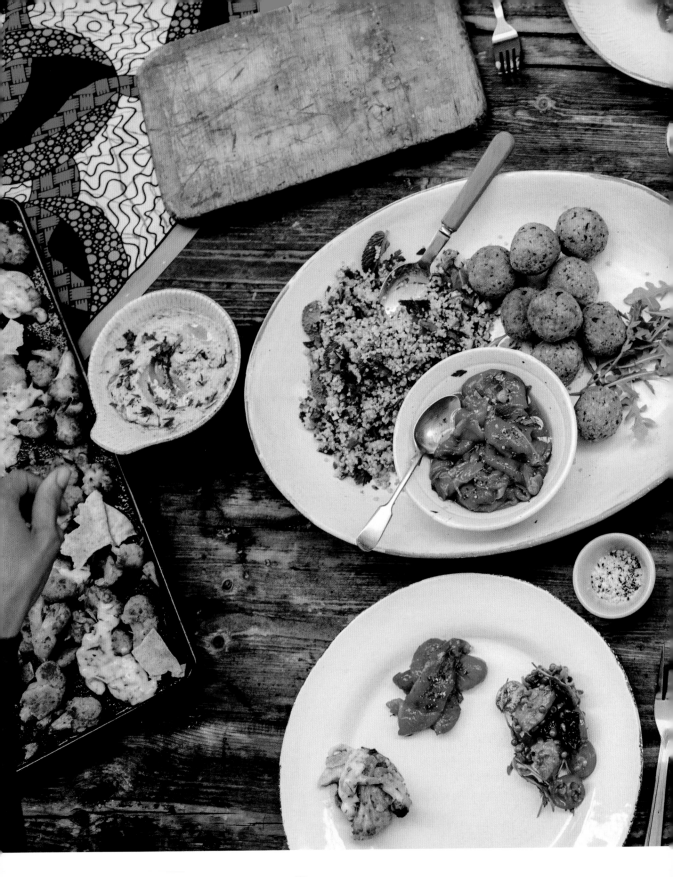

Dinner

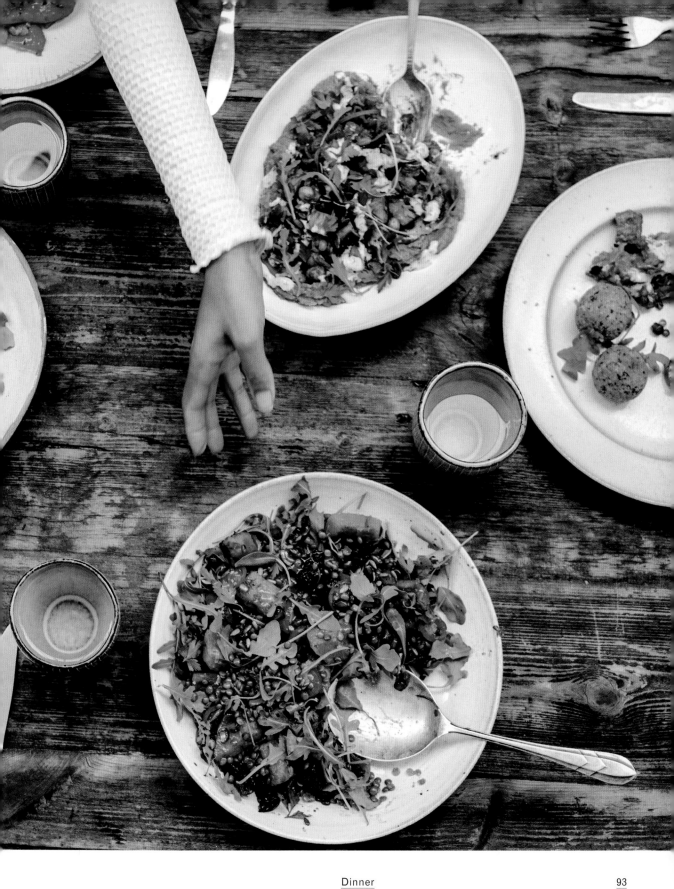

2 large raw beetroots, peeled and chopped

1 medium butternut squash, peeled, deseeded and chopped

Leaves from 2 rosemary sprigs, chopped

1 tbsp olive oil

1 tbsp maple syrup

1 × 400g tin of brown lentils, drained and rinsed

200g mixed rocket and other salad leaves

200g cherry tomatoes, quartered

4 tbsp sunflower seeds

Handful of fresh parsley, finely chopped

4 tbsp pomegranate seeds

Salt and black pepper

For the tahini vinaigrette

3 tbsp extra-virgin olive oil

1 tbsp tahini

1 tsp maple syrup

1 tsp Dijon mustard

1–2 tsp balsamic vinegar (to taste)

Roasted Beets and Butternut Squash with Tahini

A hearty salad that combines maple-glazed squash and beets with salad leaves, tomatoes and nutritious lentils, all drizzled in a creamy tahini dressing. If you're not a fan of balsamic vinegar, you can substitute it with fresh lemon juice. I like to use light tahini for a smooth dressing – I've listed a few brands I like on page 244 as some can be quite bitter.

Preheat the oven to 200°C fan.

Place the beetroot, butternut squash and rosemary in a large baking tray or roasting tin and toss in the olive oil, maple syrup and some salt and pepper until evenly coated. Spread out the vegetables in a single layer and roast in the oven for 40–50 minutes, stirring once halfway through the cooking time, until tender and slightly crisp.

Meanwhile, combine all the ingredients for the tahini vinaigrette together in a bowl, seasoning to taste with salt and pepper.

Place the lentils and salad leaves in large bowl with the cherry tomatoes and a small drizzle of the tahini vinaigrette and toss until evenly coated.

Transfer the dressed salad to a serving dish and add the still-warm roast vegetables in layers with the sunflower seeds, parsley and pomegranate seeds. Finish with a generous drizzle of vinaigrette.

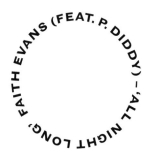

FAITH EVANS (FEAT. P. DIDDY) – 'ALL NIGHT LONG'

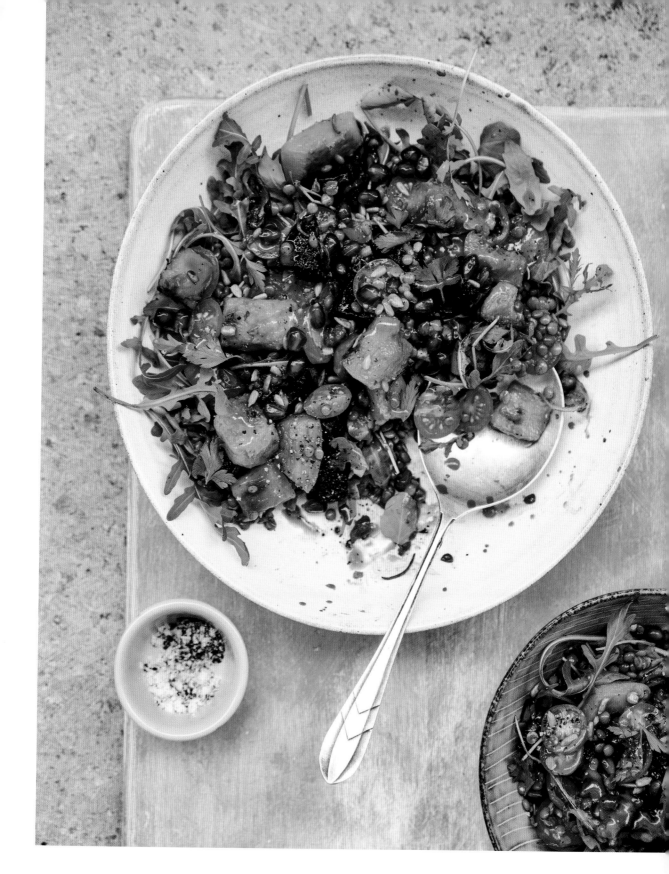

Serves 4

180g quinoa
1 head of broccoli, roughly
    chopped into florets
4 large tbsp Sun-dried
    Tomato Pesto
    (see page 121)
Salt and black pepper

To serve
Handful of mixed baby
    spinach and salad leaves
300g cherry tomatoes, halved
2 avocados, sliced
100g alfalfa sprouts
1 lemon, cut into 4 wedges

Sun-dried Tomato Pesto Quinoa Salad

Quinoa is a complete protein, so I love getting it into my recipes – but it has to be bang! Combining it with this really flavoursome sun-dried tomato pesto takes it to another level. Perfect in the summer when you want light but delicious meals.

Rinse the quinoa well under the cold tap, then add to a saucepan with double the amount of water. Season with salt and bring to the boil, then reduce the heat, cover with a lid and simmer for 10–15 minutes until the quinoa is tender and all the liquid has been absorbed. Fluff up the grains with a fork, and transfer to a bowl to cool down completely.

Meanwhile, steam the broccoli for 5 minutes and remove from the heat when slightly softened and still vibrant in colour.

Once the quinoa has cooled, mix in the sun-dried tomato pesto and steamed broccoli to combine, then season to taste with salt and pepper.

Divide the quinoa between plates and add to each a portion of mixed spinach and salad leaves, a few tomato halves, some avocado and alfalfa sprouts. Squeeze over a wedge of lemon and season with salt and pepper.

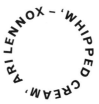

ARI LENNOX – 'WHIPPED CREAM'

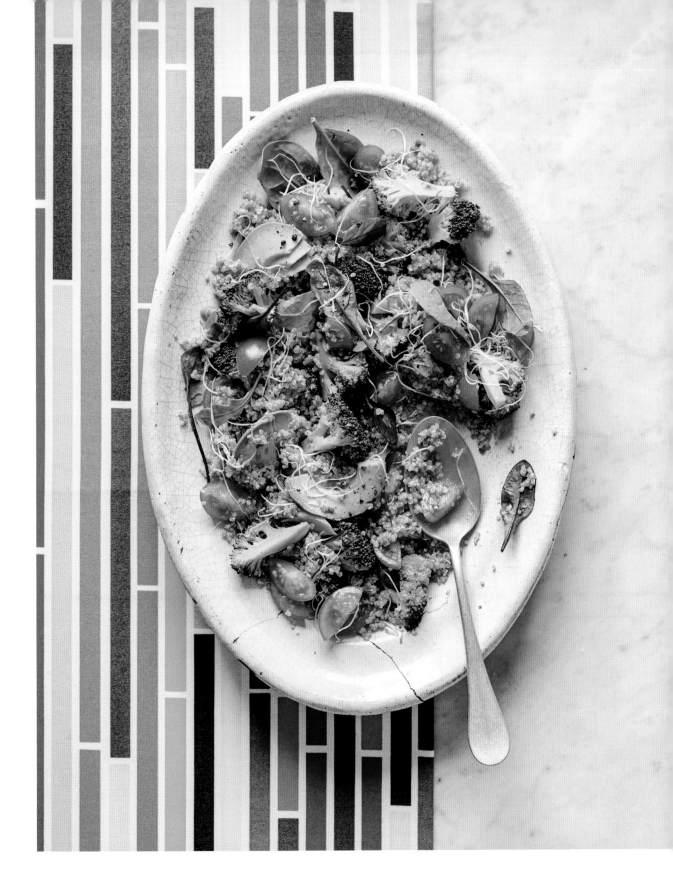

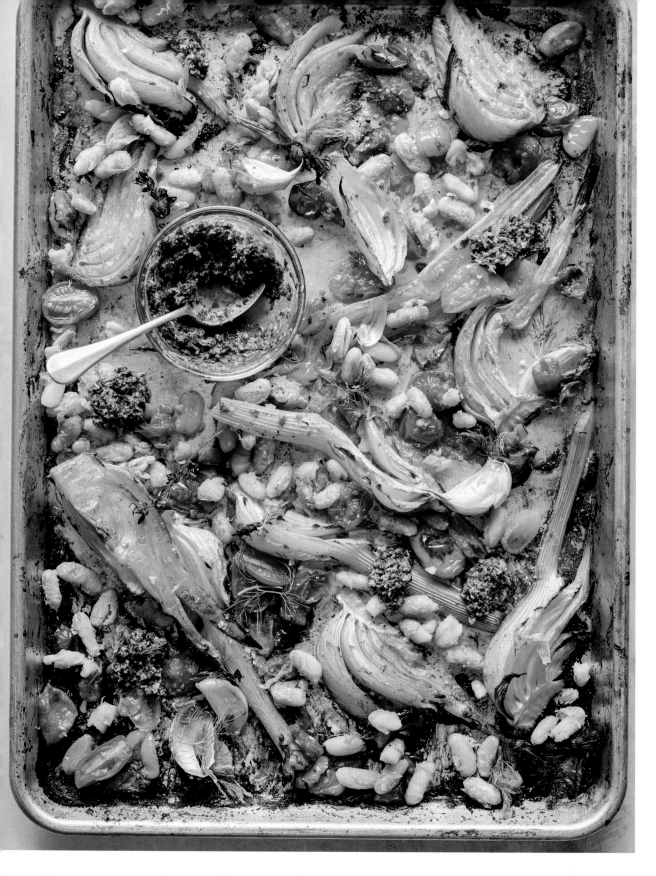

2 fennel bulbs, quartered
    lengthways, saving any
    fronds to garnish
2 garlic cloves,
    lightly crushed
250g baby plum (or cherry)
    tomatoes, halved
2 tsp harissa paste
Juice and grated zest of
    1 lemon

Leaves from 2 thyme sprigs
3–5 tbsp olive oil
1 × 400g tin of cannellini
    beans, drained and rinsed
Salt and black pepper
Handful of rocket leaves,
    to serve

For the salsa verde
½ garlic clove,
    roughly chopped
Large handful of fresh
    parsley, roughly chopped
Handful of fresh mint leaves,
    roughly chopped
1 tbsp capers
1 tsp Dijon mustard
6 tbsp extra-virgin olive oil
Juice of ½ lemon

Harissa Roast Fennel and Plum Tomatoes

Adding harissa paste is a really quick and easy way to get in tasty hot peppers and Moroccan spices to jazz up any dish. These roasted plum tomatoes and fennel pair so well with harissa and the cannellini beans and make for a warming, juicy and filling meal. They're topped with a fresh salsa verde to balance the spice. You can even turn the leftovers into a sandwich or wrap and add some lettuce or other leaves.

Preheat the oven to 200°C fan.

Place the fennel, garlic and tomatoes in a large roasting tin and add the harissa paste, lemon juice and zest, thyme and 3 tablespoons of the olive oil. Season with salt and pepper and mix everything together so that the vegetables are evenly coated.

Roast in the oven for 25 minutes, then turn the fennel pieces over to crisp up on the other side, and add the cannellini beans between the gaps in the roasting tin. Drizzle a little more olive oil on top and roast for a further 10 minutes until the fennel is soft and golden and the beans are slightly crispy.

Meanwhile, make the salsa verde by placing all the ingredients in a food processor, seasoning with salt and pepper and blitzing to a coarse paste. Alternatively, finely chop the garlic, herbs and capers and mix together in a bowl with the mustard, olive oil, lemon juice and some salt and pepper.

Serve the roasted vegetables garnished with fennel fronds (if using), with a dollop of salsa verde and a few rocket leaves.

Serves 2 as a main
or 4 as a side

1 cauliflower, broken into
    small florets and saving
    the outer leaves
1 tsp ground turmeric
1 tbsp curry powder
2 tbsp coconut oil, melted
3 poppadoms,
    plus extra to serve
Salt and black pepper
Mango chutney, to serve

**For the courgette
coconut raita**
200g unsweetened vegan
    coconut yoghurt
2 tbsp extra-virgin olive oil
¼ courgette, finely grated
Small handful of mint
    leaves, roughly chopped,
    saving some whole leaves
    to garnish

Juice and grated zest of
    1 lime (saving half the
    juice for dressing the
    cauliflower)

Curry-roasted Cauliflower with Coconut Raita

This curry-roasted cauliflower really is amazing! The combination of the aromatic spices with the soft but slightly crunchy cauliflower and the cooling courgette coconut raita is truly addictive, especially when served with a few crispy poppadoms and some mango chutney for dunking them into. This recipe would also make a fantastic side for a curry or dhal.

Preheat the oven to 200°C fan.

Place the cauliflower florets in a roasting tin with the spices, some salt and pepper and the coconut oil, then mix everything together so that the cauliflower is evenly coated. Roast in the oven for 20 minutes, then remove from the oven and mix in the cauliflower leaves, tearing up any that look too big. Place back in the oven to roast for a further 10 minutes until everything is soft and slightly charred.

Meanwhile, mix together all the raita ingredients in a bowl, season with salt and pepper and set aside.

Remove the cauliflower from the oven, add the lime juice (reserved from making the raita) and crunch the poppadoms on top. Serve with the raita, mango chutney and poppadoms and garnish with the whole mint leaves.

Dinner

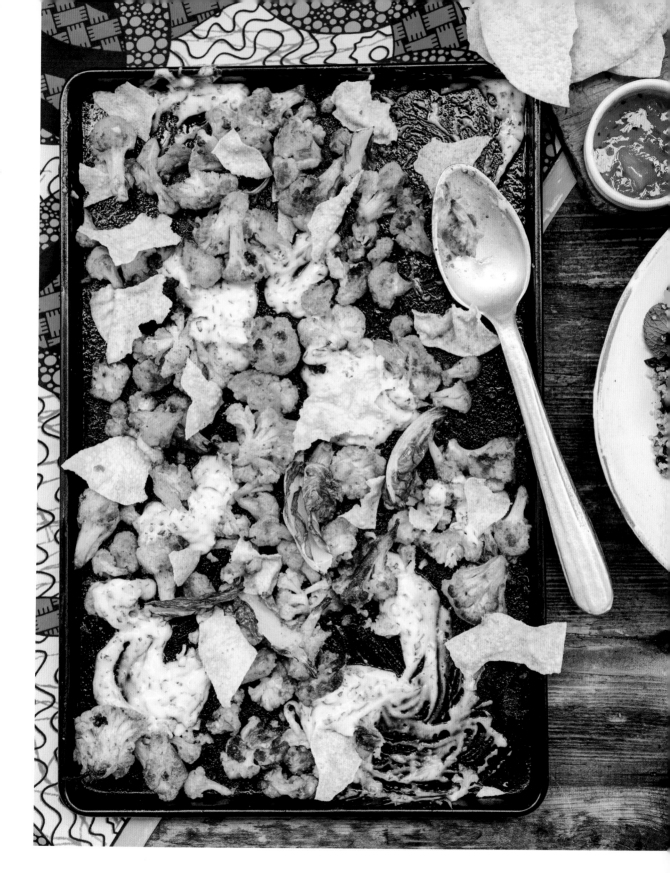

Serves 4

2 aubergines
1 tbsp vegetable oil
4 large flatbreads
    (or pitta breads)
1 quantity of Hummus
    (see page 177)
1 quantity of Tzatziki
    (see page 180)
1 red onion, finely sliced
4 tomatoes, sliced
Handful of lettuce leaves,
    roughly chopped
Handful of fresh coriander,
    roughly chopped
1 lemon, cut into 4 wedges

For the marinade

½ tsp cayenne pepper
1 tsp ground coriander
2 tbsp paprika
1 tbsp ground allspice
½ tsp ground sumac
½ tsp ground nutmeg
3 garlic cloves,
    finely chopped
2 tbsp olive oil
1 tbsp fresh lemon juice
1 tbsp finely chopped parsley
Salt and black pepper

For the mild chilli sauce

1 quantity of Roast Red
    Peppers (see page 154) or
1 × 450g jar of roasted red
    peppers in oil, drained
4 fresh medium-heat red
    chillies, deseeded and
    roughly chopped
1 tbsp fresh lemon juice
3 garlic cloves,
    roughly chopped
½ tsp sweet smoked paprika
½ tsp ground cumin
2 tbsp olive oil
1 tsp vegan
    white wine vinegar

Spiced Griddled Aubergine Kebabs and Tzatziki

An epic twist on regular kebabs, these spiced aubergines are full of flavour and have an amazing texture! I've served them in flatbreads with a cooling tzatziki, a mild chilli sauce, hummus and fresh salad. This recipe has quite a few components to it, but it is totally worth it when you put them all together. Your taste buds will be dancing, that's for sure! If you can't find vegan-friendly flatbreads (some brands add dairy), you could use pitta breads instead.

Slice the aubergines in half lengthways and then widthways into four. Slice each part into long chunks and place in a large bowl.

In a separate bowl, mix all the marinade ingredients with a sprinkling of salt and pepper. Pour the marinade all over the aubergine and use your hands to mix everything together so that the aubergines are well coated.

Next make the chilli sauce. Add the roast red peppers to a food processor with the chillies, lemon juice and garlic and then blitz into a rough sauce. Pour into a pan and add the smoked paprika, cumin and some salt and pepper. Cook over a medium heat for 6–8 minutes, stirring, until the sauce has reduced and thickened.

Transfer the sauce to a screw-top jar, pour in the olive oil and white wine vinegar, close with the lid and shake to combine. Or you can just mix it in a bowl.

Place a griddle pan (or a heavy-based frying pan) over a medium–high heat and add the vegetable oil. Once the pan is hot, add the marinated aubergine chunks and cook for 4–5 minutes until lightly chargrilled all over.

Meanwhile, toast the flatbreads in a dry non-stick frying pan over a medium heat for a couple of minutes on each side. To one side of each toasted flatbread add a layer of hummus, chilli sauce and tzatziki, then add a few aubergine chunks, followed by some red onion, tomato and lettuce. Finish with a handful of coriander and season to taste, then squeeze over a wedge of lemon and fold the flatbread over to enclose the filling.

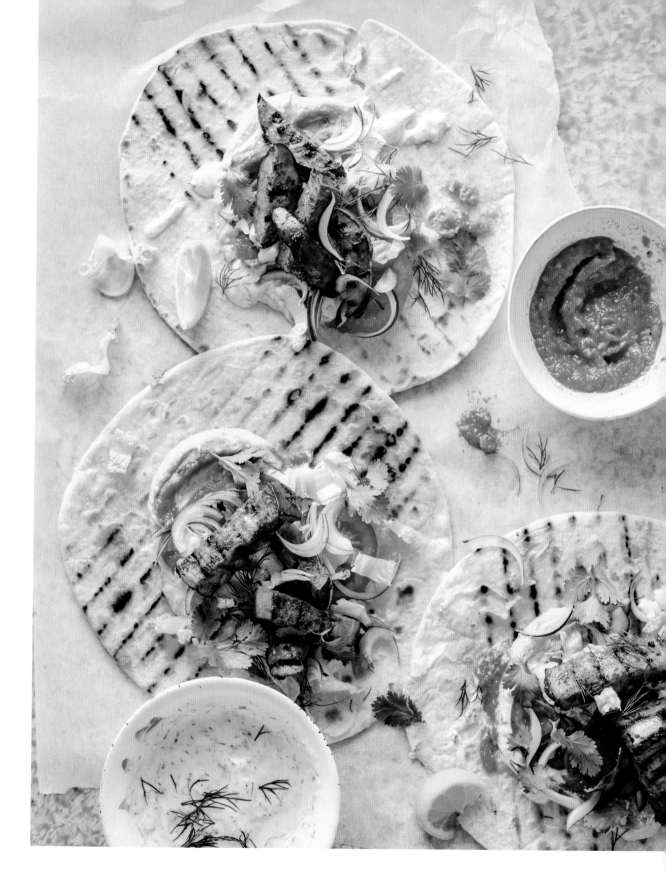

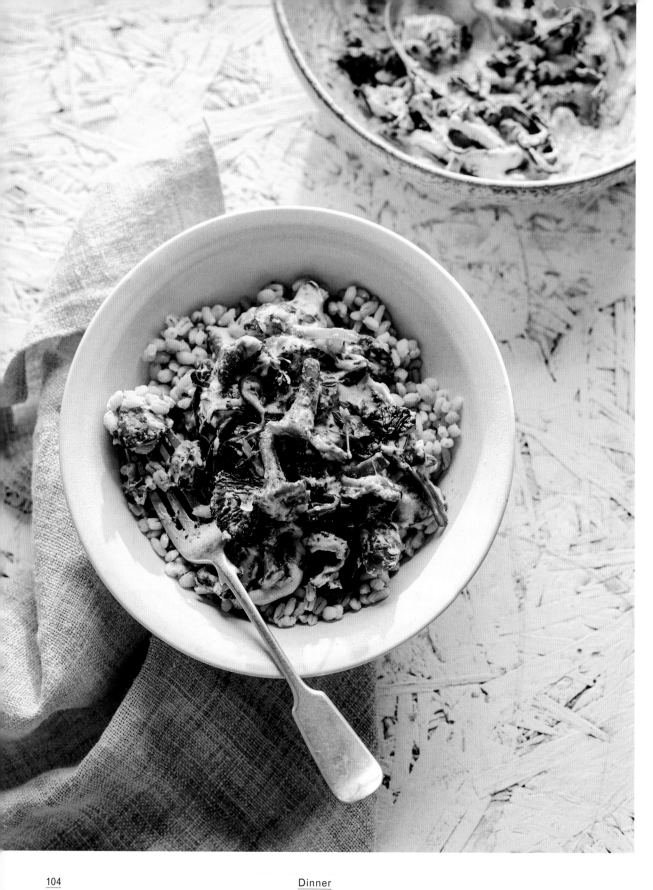

Dinner

Serves 4

350g pearl barley

For the cashew sauce
175g raw cashew nuts
2 tsp nutritional yeast
200ml water
Salt and black pepper

For the mushrooms
2 tbsp olive oil
1 large white onion,
    thinly sliced
2 garlic cloves,
    finely chopped
Leaves from 2 thyme sprigs
400g chestnut mushrooms,
    halved or quartered
    if large

Juice of ½ lemon
150ml vegetable stock
Large handful of spinach
Handful of fresh parsley,
    roughly chopped,
    plus extra to garnish

Creamy Mushrooms with Pearl Barley

A super-simple, flavoursome bowlful. Pearl barley does a really amazing job at absorbing all the flavours it's cooked in so it creates these tasty, slightly chewy mouthfuls. Pure comfort food!

Cover the cashew nuts with water and leave to soak overnight, or for a minimum of 3 hours, then drain.

Add the drained cashews, along with all the ingredients for the cashew sauce, to a high-speed blender or food processor and blend until smooth.

Meanwhile, cook the pearl barley in boiling salted water for 20 minutes until tender but not totally soft. Drain and set aside.

Place 1 tablespoon of the olive oil into a pan, add the onion and sauté over a medium–high heat for 5 minutes until softened and golden, then remove from the pan and set aside.

Add the remaining oil to the pan, followed by the garlic, thyme and mushrooms, and fry for 4–5 minutes until the mushrooms are golden. Return the onions to the pan and add the lemon juice. Pour in the cashew sauce and the vegetable stock, then bring to a gentle simmer and add the spinach and parsley. Stir for a couple of minutes to allow the fresh leaves to wilt, then season to taste with salt and pepper.

Remove from the heat and serve with the pearl barley and with extra parsley sprinkled over.

Serves 6–8

1 tbsp vegetable oil
1 red onion, diced
1 red pepper,
    deseeded and diced
4 garlic cloves,
    finely chopped
1–2 tsp chilli powder
    (to taste)
1 tsp ground coriander
1 tbsp paprika
1 tbsp ground cumin
2 × 400g tins of chopped
    tomatoes

1 × 400g tin of green lentils,
    drained and rinsed
1 × 400g tin of red kidney
    beans, drained and rinsed
1 × 400g tin of black beans,
    drained and rinsed
1 × 340g tin of sweetcorn,
    drained and rinsed
500ml vegetable stock
3 tbsp tomato purée
1 tbsp maple syrup
1 cinnamon stick
Salt and black pepper

To serve
380g brown rice
Handful of fresh coriander,
    roughly chopped
2 avocados, sliced
Vegan crème fraîche

Vegetable Chilli

An absolute staple in my kitchen! This super-hearty, simple chilli is a saviour when I want to make something nutritious and filling without too much fuss – just throw it all in one large pot! A definite go-to recipe for guests too as it always goes down well.

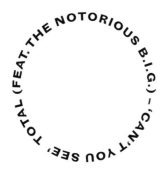

TOTAL (FEAT. THE NOTORIOUS B.I.G.) – 'CAN'T YOU SEE'

Heat the vegetable oil in a large, heavy-based saucepan or shallow frying pan. Add the onion and red pepper and sauté over a medium heat for 6–7 minutes until softened and beginning to brown. Add the garlic and ground spices and sauté for 5 minutes. Stir frequently and add 1–2 tablespoons of water to the mixture if the spices begin to stick to the pan.

Pour in the tinned tomatoes, lentils, beans and sweetcorn, then add the vegetable stock. Add the tomato purée, maple syrup and cinnamon stick and mix in well, seasoning with salt and pepper.

Cover the pan with a lid and bring to the boil, then reduce the heat and simmer over a medium heat for 20 minutes. Remove the lid and simmer for another 10 minutes until thickened.

Meanwhile, cook the rice. Thoroughly rinse under the cold tap until the water runs clear, to remove any excess starch, then place in a saucepan with double the quantity of water and a good pinch of salt. Stir the rice in the water and bring to the boil, then cover the pan with a lid, reduce the heat to low and simmer for 30 minutes, or until the rice is tender and the water has been absorbed. Remove the pan from the heat and leave to stand, still covered with the lid, for 5 minutes, then remove the lid and fluff up the grains of rice with a fork.

Serve the chilli with the rice and garnish with the coriander, avocado and a dollop of vegan crème fraîche.

Dinner

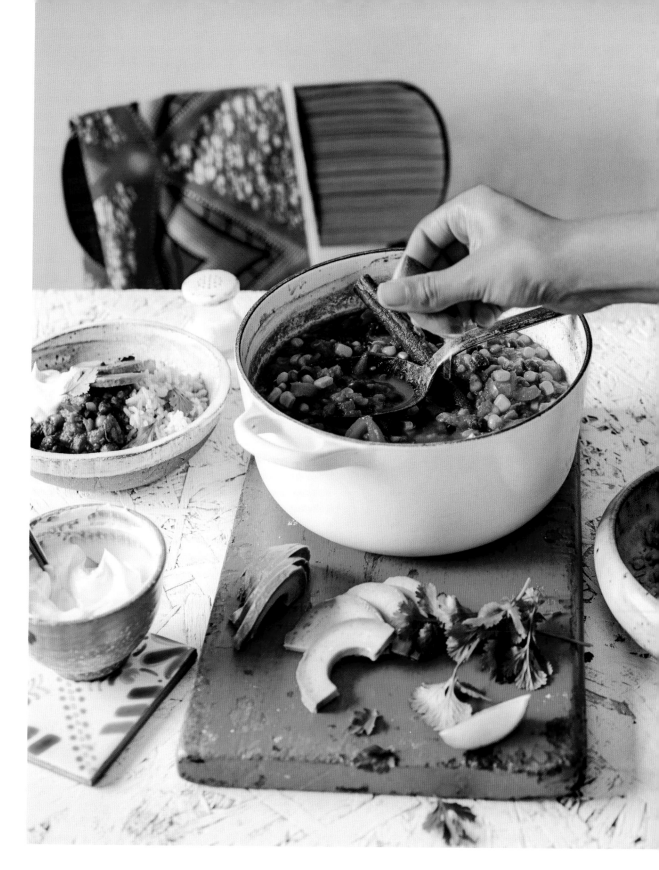

Serves 4

1 head of broccoli, roughly
    chopped into florets
4 garlic cloves,
    finely chopped
2 red onions, roughly sliced
400g cherry tomatoes, halved
3 tbsp olive oil
500g dried linguine
100g spinach,
    roughly chopped
Salt and black pepper
Handful of fresh parsley,
    finely chopped, to garnish
Extra-virgin olive oil,
    for drizzling

For the cashew sauce
120g raw cashew nuts
240ml water
2 tbsp nutritional yeast
1 tbsp fresh lemon juice
1 tsp garlic granules

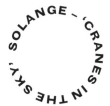

Creamy Linguine with Roast Vegetables

This recipe is guaranteed to be a big hit with all pasta lovers. Cashew nuts flavoured with garlic and nutritional yeast make a super-smooth and creamy pasta sauce that is so simple to prepare. Combine with roasted cherry tomatoes, broccoli and red onions and top with fresh parsley and black pepper for a truly comforting dinner.

Cover the cashew nuts with water and leave to soak overnight, or for a minimum of 3 hours, then drain.

Preheat the oven to 180°C fan.

Place the broccoli, garlic, onions and tomatoes in a roasting tin. Spread the vegetables out evenly in the tin, then drizzle with the olive oil and sprinkle with salt and pepper. Place in the oven to roast for 15 minutes, then remove from the oven, toss the vegetables in the tin and roast for another 10–15 minutes until they are tender and lightly caramelised.

Meanwhile, place the drained cashews and all the other ingredients for the cashew sauce in a high-speed blender or a food processor, season with salt and pepper and blend until smooth.

Cook the linguine in a large saucepan of boiling salted water according to the packet instructions or until al dente, then drain in a colander, reserving a little of the cooking water.

Return the cooked pasta to the pan and set over a low heat, add the roast vegetables and spinach and fold together well, letting the spinach wilt in the pasta. Pour in the cashew sauce and mix to combine. If the sauce is too thick, add a bit of the reserved pasta-cooking water to loosen it.

Remove from heat, then divide between bowls, sprinkle with parsley and add a drizzle of extra-virgin olive oil and a grind of black pepper.

Dinner

Serves 4

500g dried spaghetti
Extra-virgin olive oil,
    for drizzling
Handful of parsley, roughly
    chopped, to garnish
1 quantity of Herby
    Macadamia Crunch
    (see page 151)

**For the vegetable
Bolognese sauce**
1 tbsp olive oil
1 red onion, diced
4 garlic cloves,
    finely chopped
2 medium carrots,
    peeled and diced
2 celery sticks,
    finely chopped
1 aubergine,
    cut into small chunks
1 tbsp dried oregano

Leaves from
    1 rosemary sprig,
    chopped
2 bay leaves
2 × 400g tins of
    plum tomatoes
200g dried green lentils
500ml vegetable stock
1 tbsp sun-dried
    tomato purée
1 tbsp brown miso paste
1 tsp maple syrup (optional)
Salt and black pepper

Vegetable Spaghetti Bolognese

An Italian family classic that tastes just as good made only with vegetables. The miso paste adds a punch of umami flavour that makes this vegan sauce super tasty, while aubergines and lentils add texture and keep it filling, though you could swap them for vegan mince, if you prefer.

First make the vegetable Bolognese sauce. Pour the oil into a large saucepan, add the onion and sauté over a medium heat for 4–5 minutes until soft. Add the garlic, carrots, celery, aubergine, oregano, rosemary and bay leaves and cook, stirring frequently, for another 10 minutes until the aubergine has browned slightly and the carrots and celery are tender.

Pour in the tinned tomatoes and lentils, followed by the vegetable stock, then add the sun-dried tomato purée, miso paste and maple syrup (if using), and season with salt and pepper. Mix everything together well, then bring to a simmer, cover with a lid and cook for 30 minutes, then remove the lid and simmer for another 10 minutes until the lentils are cooked through. Taste and add more salt and pepper if needed. Remove the bay leaves.

Place the spaghetti in a large saucepan of boiling salted water and cook according to the packet instructions until al dente, then drain in a colander.

Toss the cooked spaghetti in the vegetable Bolognese sauce, then drizzle with a little extra-virgin olive oil, garnish with the parsley and sprinkle with black pepper and the herby macadamia crunch to serve.

500g dried spaghetti

**For the juna
(jackfruit tuna)**
1 × 400g tin of jackfruit,
    drained and rinsed
3 tbsp soy sauce
    (or coconut aminos)
1 tbsp fresh lemon juice
2 tbsp nori flakes

For the tomato sauce
1 tbsp olive oil
1 red onion, finely diced
4 garlic cloves,
    finely chopped
1 tsp dried oregano
1 tsp dried basil
2 × 400g tins of
    cherry tomatoes
1 tbsp balsamic vinegar
1–2 tsp maple syrup
    (optional, for sweetness)
Handful of mixed olives,
    pitted and chopped
Handful of capers
Salt and black pepper

To serve
Handful of fresh parsley,
    chopped
Handful of Herby Macadamia
    Crunch (see page 151)
4 tbsp extra-virgin olive oil

Juna Pasta

Tuna pasta covered in cheese was pretty much the meal that got me through university. I wanted to devise a version of it that evoked the original dish but without using tuna or cheese, so I came up with this recipe, made with jackfruit. It still takes me right back to my uni days but tastes much more delicious! To make it soy-free, simply substitute coconut aminos for the soy sauce. The song choice is a song that came out way before I studied at university, but it got some serious airtime in my room at uni with my huge speakers – apologies to my flatmates for the heavy bass.

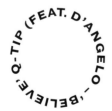

First prepare the juna. In a bowl, using clean hands or a fork, break the jackfruit into small pieces, removing any tough stems, the stir in the soy sauce, lemon juice and nori flakes. Mix well to combine, then cover the bowl with a plate and set aside while you prepare the rest of the dish.

Pour the olive oil into a deep saucepan set over a medium heat, add the red onion and sauté for about 7 minutes until softened. Stir in the garlic, dried oregano and basil and cook for 3–4 minutes, stirring from time to time, then add the tinned tomatoes and balsamic vinegar. Season with salt and pepper, then bring to a simmer and cook for 15 minutes, stirring occasionally. Check the flavour and add 1 teaspoon of the maple syrup if needed.

Mix the juna into the tomato sauce with the olives and capers. Bring the sauce back up to the boil, then reduce the heat to low and cook for another 15 minutes, stirring occasionally. Taste for seasoning, adding more maple syrup and salt and pepper if needed.

Meanwhile, cook the spaghetti in a saucepan of boiling salted water according to the packet instructions until it is al dente. Drain in a colander and then tip the spaghetti into the pan with the tomato sauce.

Stir the spaghetti into the sauce, then divide between plates or bowls and serve each garnished with the parsley, herby macadamia crunch, a grind of pepper and a tablespoon of extra-virgin olive oil drizzled over.

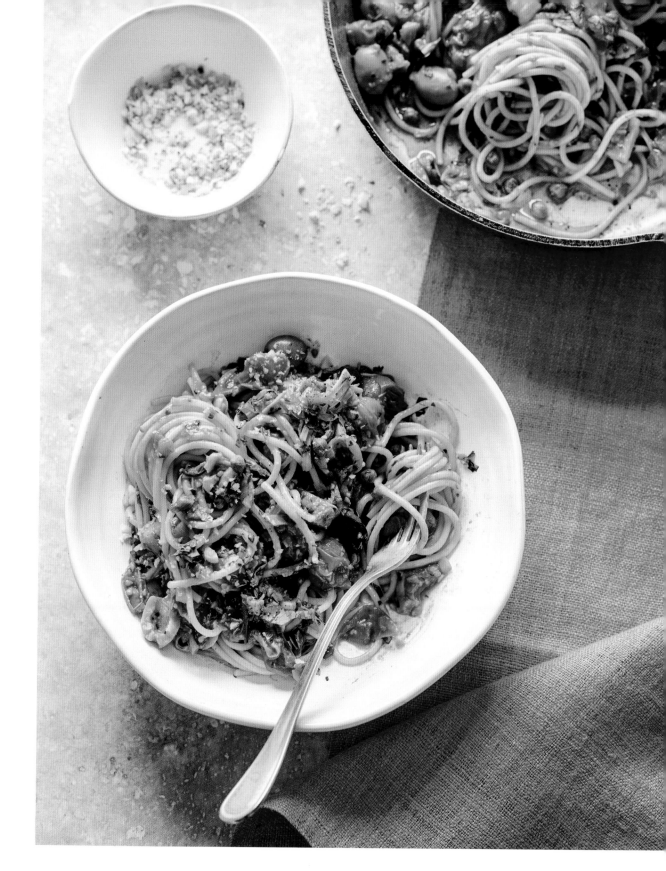

Serves 6

1 large aubergine,
    cut lengthways
    into 5mm slices
1 large courgette,
    cut lengthways
    into 5mm slices
2 tbsp olive oil
1 quantity of Herby
    Macadamia Crunch
    (see page 151)
Extra-virgin olive oil,
    for drizzling
Mixed salad leaves, to serve

For the cashew sauce
240g raw cashew nuts,
    soaked overnight
2 tbsp nutritional yeast
2 tbsp fresh lemon juice
2 tsp garlic granules
Handful of basil leaves

For the tomato sauce
1 tbsp olive oil
1 onion, finely diced
3 garlic cloves, finely chopped
1 tsp dried oregano
1 tsp dried basil
120g shiitake mushrooms,
    roughly chopped

2 × 400g tins of
    chopped tomatoes
1 × 400g tin of brown lentils,
    drained and rinsed
1 tbsp tomato purée
1 tbsp balsamic vinegar
1 tbsp brown miso paste
    (optional)
1 tsp maple syrup (optional)
Handful of parsley,
    roughly chopped,
    plus extra to garnish
Salt and black pepper

**You will need a 2-litre
gratin dish**

Creamy Cashew and Vegetable No-pasta Lasagne

A vegetable lasagne made by layering courgettes and aubergines with a tasty tomato sauce and a creamy cashew cheese sauce. A wheat-free twist on regular lasagne, it's both comforting and full of flavour – you won't feel you're missing out. A fantastic and delicious way to get the entire family indulging in their vegetables!

MARVIN GAYE – 'HEARD IT THROUGH THE GRAPEVINE'

Preheat the oven to 180°C fan. Place the aubergine and courgette slices on a baking tray, spreading them out in a single layer and using two trays if needed, drizzle with the olive oil, season with salt and pepper and roast in the oven for 15 minutes. Meanwhile, make the tomato sauce.

Pour the oil into a large deep saucepan set over a medium heat, then add the onion and sauté until lightly browned. Stir in the garlic and dried herbs, followed by the mushrooms and cook for another 5 minutes until these start to brown. Add the tomatoes, lentils, tomato purée, balsamic vinegar and miso (if using). Season with salt and pepper, then bring to a simmer and cook, uncovered, for 15 minutes, stirring occasionally, until thickened. Check the flavour and add the maple syrup if needed. Remove from the heat and stir in the parsley.

Put all the ingredients for the cashew sauce except the basil into a blender or food processor with 240ml water. Season and blitz until smooth. Add more salt and pepper to taste, and more water, bit by bit, if needed, to reach the desired consistency. Stir in the basil.

To assemble, spread a quarter of the tomato sauce over the bottom of the gratin dish. Add the aubergines in a single layer, followed by a layer of tomato sauce. Then add half of the cashew sauce, followed by more tomato sauce, then a layer of courgettes. For the top, add the rest of the tomato sauce, then swirl in the remaining cashew sauce and sprinkle with the herby macadamia crunch. Bake for 15–20 minutes, keeping an eye on the layer of nuts, until browned. Drizzle with olive oil, garnish with parsley and serve with the leaves.

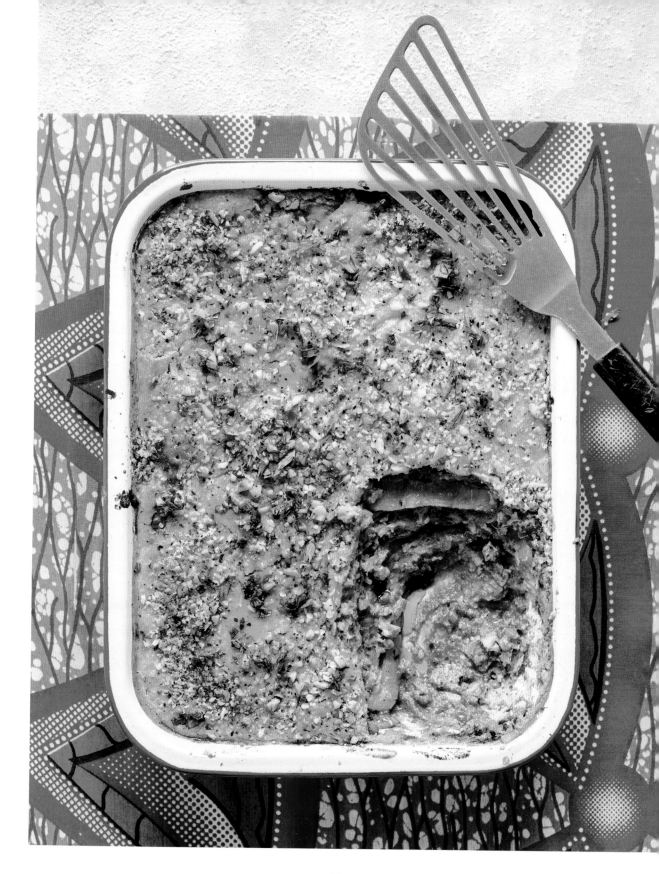

Serves 4

800g dried lasagne sheets
1 quantity of Herby
   Macadamia Crunch
   (see page 151)

For the ragù
1 tbsp olive oil
1 onion, finely diced
1 carrot, peeled and
   finely chopped
1 celery stick, finely chopped
4 garlic cloves,
   finely chopped

Leaves from 1 rosemary
   sprig, chopped
1 tsp dried oregano
1 tsp dried basil
2 × 400g tins of
   chopped tomatoes
240g vegan mince
1 tbsp sun-dried
   tomato purée
1 tbsp balsamic vinegar
1 tbsp brown miso paste
1 tsp maple syrup (optional)

For the white sauce
4 tbsp vegan butter
3 tbsp plain flour
480ml soy milk
½ tsp ground nutmeg
1 tbsp nutritional yeast
Salt and black pepper

**You will need a 2-litre
gratin dish**

Vegan Lasagne

A comfort-food classic! Combining a creamy vegan béchamel with a rich vegetable ragù, it's hard to not keep going back for more. You can make this with your choice of vegan mince, if you prefer, or stick to using vegetables (see opposite). You could also add your favourite vegan cheese on the top, instead of using the herby macadamia crunch, but the white sauce gives enough creamy comfort for me.

To make the ragù, heat the olive oil in a large saucepan, add the onion, carrot, celery and garlic, followed by the rosemary, oregano and basil, and sauté over a low heat for 7–10 minutes until the vegetables have softened.

Pour in the tinned tomatoes and vegan mince and add the sun-dried tomato purée, balsamic vinegar, miso paste and maple syrup (if using). Mix well to combine, then bring to a simmer and cook on a low heat for 15 minutes.

Meanwhile, make the white sauce. Melt the butter in a pan over a low heat and add the flour, whisking to combine and then cook for 2 minutes. Remove from the heat and gradually whisk in the soy milk to make a loose sauce. Season with the nutmeg, nutritional yeast and some salt and pepper to taste, then return to a gentle heat and whisk constantly until the sauce thickens.

Preheat the oven to 180°C fan.

CARLTON – 'SHE'S A BAD MAMA JAMA', CARL

Layer up the lasagne in the gratin dish, starting with a third of the ragù, then a layer of lasagne sheets and a third of the white sauce. Repeat twice, adding the white sauce as the top layer, then sprinkle the herby macadamia crunch over the top.

Bake in the oven for 40–45 minutes, or according to the lasagne packet instructions, until piping hot and lightly browned. Keep an eye on the dish during cooking to make sure the layer of nuts on top doesn't burn.

VEGETABLE OPTION

Replace the vegan mince with 1 medium aubergine and 1 courgette, both diced, and a 400g tin of brown lentils, drained and rinsed. Add the aubergine and courgette to the pan after cooking the other vegetables for 7–10 minutes and cook for another 5–7 minutes until lightly browned. Add the lentils to the pan at the same time as the tinned tomatoes and then continue to prepare the lasagne as above.

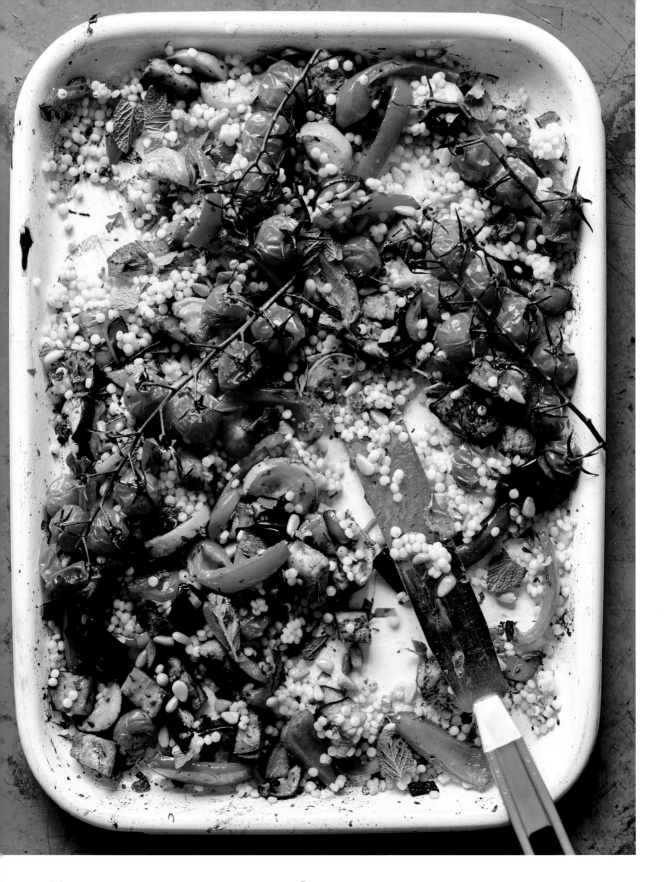

Dinner

Serves 4

1 large aubergine, chopped
    into small cubes
1 courgette, halved
    lengthways and chopped
    into crescents 5mm thick
2 red peppers, deseeded
    and sliced
2 tbsp olive oil
2 tsp dried oregano

2 tsp dried parsley
Leaves from 2 thyme sprigs
5 garlic cloves,
    finely chopped
1 red onion, roughly chopped
200g cherry tomatoes
200g giant couscous
Juice of 1 lemon
Salt and black pepper

To serve
50g pine nuts
Handful of fresh parsley,
    finely chopped
Handful of fresh mint leaves,
    finely chopped

One-tray Roast Vegetables with Couscous and Herbs

Roasting vegetables is one of my favourite ways both to clear out the fridge and get all my veggies for the day in a really tasty hit. Enjoy the ease of throwing them all in a single tray and popping them straight in the oven, then mixing with couscous for a super-simple meal.

Preheat the oven to 180°C fan.

Place the aubergine, courgette and red peppers in a roasting tin and mix with the olive oil, dried herbs, fresh thyme, garlic and red onion. Season with salt and pepper and spread out evenly in the roasting tin, then cover with a baking sheet and pop in the oven to roast for 20 minutes.

Remove the vegetables from the oven, add the cherry tomatoes and toss everything together, then return the roasting tin to the oven to cook, uncovered, for another 20 minutes until all the vegetables are tender, golden and crispy at the edges.

If you'd like the pine nuts to be toasted, scatter them over a baking tray and toast in the oven for 5–6 minutes, tossing them from time to time and keeping a close eye on them so that they don't burn.

Meanwhile, cook the couscous according to the packet instructions, then add to the roasting tin with the lemon juice and mix in with the roasted vegetables. Serve sprinkled with the parsley, mint and pine nuts.

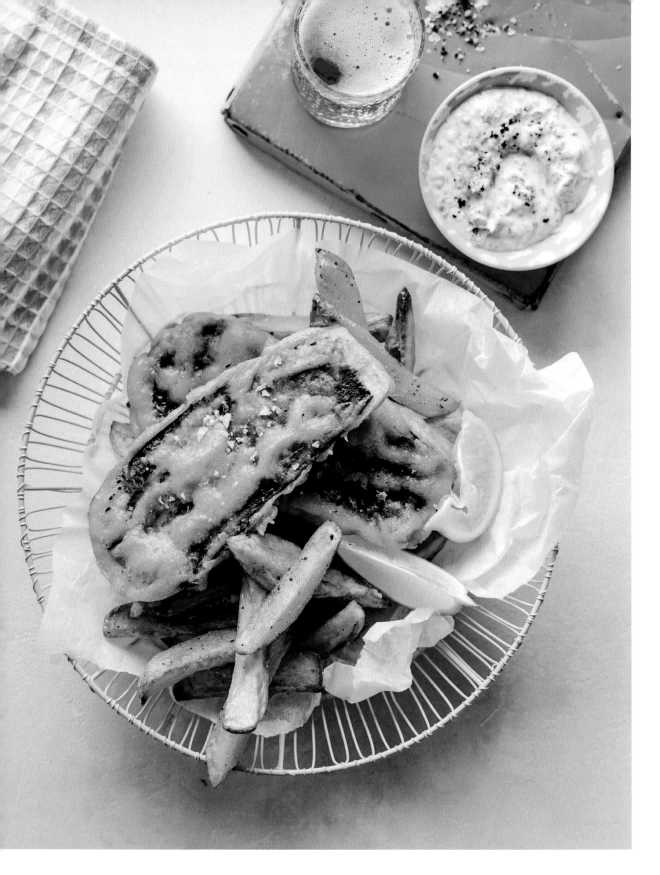

Dinner

Serves 4

2 aubergines	**For the batter**	**For the chips**
2 tbsp fresh lemon juice	100g plain flour	6 floury potatoes
2 tbsp soy sauce	75ml sparkling water	(such as Maris Piper)
(or coconut aminos)	75ml vegan beer	2 tbsp olive oil
Sunflower oil, for deep-	1 tsp baking powder	Sea salt flakes, plus extra
frying	½ tsp ground turmeric	to serve
3–4 nori sheets	½ tsp onion powder	
1 quantity of Tartare Sauce	½ tsp garlic granules	
(see page 191), to serve	Salt and black pepper	

Beer-battered Aubergine and Chips

Growing up in the UK meant that fish and chip shops were never too far away. At one point in my childhood, Friday-night fish and chips became a bit of a tradition. Admittedly I was only interested in the chips, but guess what – if you're the same, you don't have to let that go, because this fish-free version is so, so delicious! Mixed with nori sheets and soy sauce for sea flavours and fried until crispy in a light beer batter, the aubergines provide great texture and are served with chips and a vegan tartare sauce to dip into for all the Friday-night feels.

Peel and cut the potatoes lengthways into chips roughly 1cm thick, then rinse in plenty of cold water to remove any excess starch. Ideally, leave the potatoes to soak in a bowl of cold water for a few hours or overnight.

Preheat the oven to 200°C fan.

Pat the chips dry with a clean tea towel, then place on a baking tray and toss with the olive oil and some sea salt. Spread the chips in a single layer, then bake in the oven for about 45 minutes, turning every so often. Once the chips are golden, remove from the oven.

While the chips are cooking, mix all the batter ingredients in a large bowl, season with salt and pepper and whisk until smooth. Peel the aubergines and cut lengthways into 1cm-thick slices, then season with pepper.

Pour enough sunflower oil into a large, deep heavy-based saucepan to fill it no more than two-thirds full and heat the oil until it reaches 190°C on a food thermometer. Alternatively, drop in a cube of bread and, if it cooks in 30–40 seconds, the oil will be hot enough.

Continued on the next page

Place an aubergine slice on one of the nori sheets, near the edge, and cut around the aubergine. Repeat until the nori sheets have been cut into enough slices to cover one side of each aubergine slice. Mix the lemon and soy in a small bowl. Brush one side of the aubergine with a little of the lemon mixture then place a nori sheet on top. The lemon mixture should help the nori sheet stick to the aubergine.

Using a pair of tongs, pick up a nori-covered aubergine slice at one end and dip it into the batter with the nori-sheet side facing up. Use a spoon to coat the nori side with batter.

Still using the tongs, carefully place the batter-coated aubergine slice in the oil, and repeat with the other slices, coating them in the batter and placing them in the hot oil one at a time. You may need to cook them in batches, depending on the size of your pan. Cook for 4 minutes until the batter is crisp and golden, then remove with a slotted spoon and transfer to a baking tray lined with kitchen paper to drain.

Serve the battered aubergine slices with the chips and tartare sauce and a sprinkling of sea salt flakes.

500g dried spaghetti
Extra-virgin olive oil,
    for drizzling
Handful of fresh parsley,
    roughly chopped,
    to garnish

For the sun-dried tomato pesto
30g whole almonds
4 garlic cloves,
    roughly chopped
240g sun-dried tomatoes
    from a jar, drained
    and rinsed

30g fresh basil leaves,
    roughly chopped
2 tbsp nutritional yeast
1 tbsp balsamic vinegar
60ml extra-virgin olive oil
Salt and black pepper

Sun-dried Tomato Pesto Pasta

Sun-dried tomatoes, roasted almonds, garlic, herbs and extra-virgin olive oil are combined to make this rich-tasting pesto. Mix it with your favourite type of pasta (mine's spaghetti) and top with fresh parsley for a super-flavoursome meal. This pesto also goes well in sandwiches, or mixed into quinoa for a sustaining salad (see page 96).

First prepare the pesto. If the sun-dried tomatoes seem a bit tough, you can soften them by leaving them to sit in a bowl of warm water for 15 minutes before making the pesto.

Toast the almonds in a dry, heavy-based frying pan over a medium heat for 2–3 minutes until they begin to brown and give off a rich aroma. Toss regularly as they can burn very quickly, so you'll need to keep a close eye on them throughout. Remove the almonds from the pan to allow them to cool, then add them to a food processor and blitz into little pieces.

Add the rest of the pesto ingredients to the food processor and pulse into a coarse paste. Add salt and pepper to taste and pulse again.

Place the spaghetti in a large saucepan of boiling salted water and cook according to the packet instructions until al dente, then drain in a colander.

Return the drained spaghetti to the pan and toss with the pesto, then drizzle with a little extra-virgin olive oil, garnish with the parsley and grind over some black pepper to serve.

GOLDLINK – 'MEDITATION'

Serves 4

320g dried rice noodles
1 tbsp coconut oil
1 shallot, finely chopped
1 red pepper, deseeded
    and finely sliced
1 tbsp grated fresh root ginger
4 Kaffir lime leaves, torn
400ml coconut milk
600ml vegetable stock
2 tbsp vegan fish sauce
    (to make your own,
    see page 193)
1 tbsp soy sauce
1 tbsp coconut sugar
200g bok choy
Handful of Thai basil leaves

For the Thai red curry paste

6 dried red chillies, deseeded
    and soaked until tender
10 garlic cloves, chopped
Thumb-sized piece of fresh
    root ginger, peeled and
    roughly chopped
2 lemongrass stalks, tough
    outer leaves removed,
    roughly chopped
Stalks from a handful
    of fresh coriander
½ tsp ground coriander
½ tsp ground cumin
1 shallot, roughly chopped
Salt and black pepper

To serve

2 spring onions, chopped
Leaves from a handful
    of fresh coriander,
    roughly chopped
2 mild fresh red chillies,
    deseeded and
    finely chopped
200g bean sprouts
2 limes, each cut into
    4 wedges

Red Thai Curry Noodles

The curry paste in this recipe is bursting with authentic Thai flavours. Mixed in with coconut milk, root ginger, rice noodles, crunchy bean sprouts, red peppers, coriander and lime juice, it makes a dish that is both cosy and comforting yet fresh and fragrant. I especially love making it when I'm feeling a bit under the weather. The garlic, ginger and chilli warm me up from the inside and clear my sinuses. If you don't have vegan fish sauce handy, add an extra tablespoon of soy sauce.

Place all the ingredients for the Thai red curry paste in a food processor and pulse into a coarse paste, seasoning with salt and pepper. Alternatively, use a pestle and mortar to break down the ingredients.

Cook the rice noodles in a large saucepan of boiling salted water according to the packet instructions, then drain in a colander.

Melt the coconut oil in a large pan or wok set over a medium–high heat and add the shallot and red pepper. Cook, stirring occasionally, for 5 minutes, then stir in the Thai red curry paste, the ginger and Kaffir lime leaves and cook for 1 minute or until fragrant.

Pour in the coconut milk with the vegetable stock, then add the vegan fish sauce, soy sauce and coconut sugar. Bring to the boil, then reduce the heat and cook for 10 minutes, stirring occasionally and adding salt and pepper to taste, if needed.

Add the bok choy and cooked noodles, mix in well and cook for 3 minutes, then remove from the heat and stir in the Thai basil.

Serve in bowls, sprinkled with the spring onions, coriander, chillies, bean sprouts and lime wedges.

Serves 4

500g dried wide flat
  rice noodles
1 tbsp peanut oil
5 shallots, finely chopped
4 spring onions,
  roughly chopped
4 garlic cloves,
  finely chopped
2 fresh red chillies, deseeded
Thumb-sized piece
  of fresh root ginger,
  peeled and grated
4 Chinese chives,
  roughly snipped
100g bean sprouts

Juice of 1 lime
1 tbsp chilli flakes
Salt

For the sauce
4 tbsp vegan fish sauce
  (to make your own,
  see page 193)
1 tbsp soy sauce
  (or coconut aminos)
2 tsp tamarind paste
3 tbsp coconut sugar
1 tbsp vegan
  rice wine vinegar

To serve
Handful of fresh coriander,
  roughly chopped
1 lime, cut into 4 wedges
50g unsalted
  roasted peanuts,
  roughly chopped

Pad Thai

Inspired by the Thai street-food staple, this noodle stir-fry combines a sweet–savoury sauce with flat rice noodles and crunchy bean sprouts. Forget about getting a take-out when you can make this super-tasty vegan version at home. If you're in a rush and don't have any vegan fish sauce handy, you can skip it and substitute with 2 tablespoons of soy sauce (or coconut aminos or tamari), but the fish sauce does make it extra flavoursome.

Place the rice noodles in a pan of boiling salted water and cook according to the packet instructions, then drain and set aside.

In a bowl, mix together the fish sauce, soy sauce, tamarind paste, coconut sugar and rice wine vinegar, combining well to create the sauce.

Heat the peanut oil in a wok or large frying pan. Once hot, add the shallots, spring onions, garlic, chilli and ginger and stir-fry over a medium–high heat for 1–2 minutes.

Add the Chinese chives and half the bean sprouts and cook for 2 minutes, stirring occasionally. Pour in the sauce and add the noodles, lime juice and chilli flakes. Stir well to coat everything in the sauce and then cook for 2 minutes.

To serve, divide between bowls and garnish with the coriander, lime wedges, a sprinkling of roasted peanuts and the remaining spring onions and bean sprouts.

Serves 4

1 tbsp vegetable oil
1 onion, finely chopped
½–1 tsp cayenne pepper
    (to taste)
1 tbsp ground turmeric
1 tbsp paprika
1 tbsp Madras curry powder
1 tbsp ground cumin
3 garlic cloves,
    finely chopped

Thumb-sized piece of fresh
    root ginger, peeled and
    grated or finely chopped
2 medium carrots, peeled
    and cut small chunks
2 medium all-purpose
    potatoes (such as
    Désirée), peeled and
    cut into small chunks
2 × 400g tins of chickpeas,
    drained and rinsed
500ml vegetable stock
Salt and black pepper
Handful of fresh parsley,
    roughly chopped,
    to garnish

To serve
4 Dhalpuri Rotis
    (see page 166)
1 quantity of Fried Plantains
    (see page 174)
1 quantity of Red Cabbage
    Slaw (see page 155)

Caribbean Channa

In the 1800s, huge numbers of Indians were taken to Caribbean islands to work on sugar cane plantations. As such, a lot of West Indian recipes are largely influenced by India, especially in Trinidad where you'll find Trini doubles, chutneys and popular Indian seasonings, as well as comforting channa recipes like this one (basically a chickpea curry). Chickpeas combined with potatoes and carrots and a delicious blend of spices make this both hearty and full of flavour. It's perfect with the Dhalpuri Rotis on page 166, and for a feast, I love to serve it with fried plantains and coleslaw too, for a range of mouth-watering tastes and textures. For less heat, stick to ½ teaspoon of cayenne pepper.

Pour the vegetable oil into a large saucepan, add the onion and sauté over a medium heat for 5–6 minutes until softened and lightly browned. Add the spices and some salt and pepper, followed by the garlic and ginger, and cook for another 5 minutes until the garlic has softened.

Tip the carrots, potatoes and chickpeas into the pan and mix well to coat in the spiced onion mixture. Pour in the stock and stir everything together well, then cover the pan with a lid and bring to the boil. Reduce the heat and cook for about 30 minutes until the potatoes and carrots are tender, then remove the lid and simmer for another few minutes until thickened. The potatoes should help thicken the curry too. Taste and add more salt and pepper if needed.

Once cooked, remove from the heat and garnish with the chopped parsley. Serve the channa with the rotis, fried plantains and red cabbage slaw.

NINA SIMONE – 'BALTIMORE'

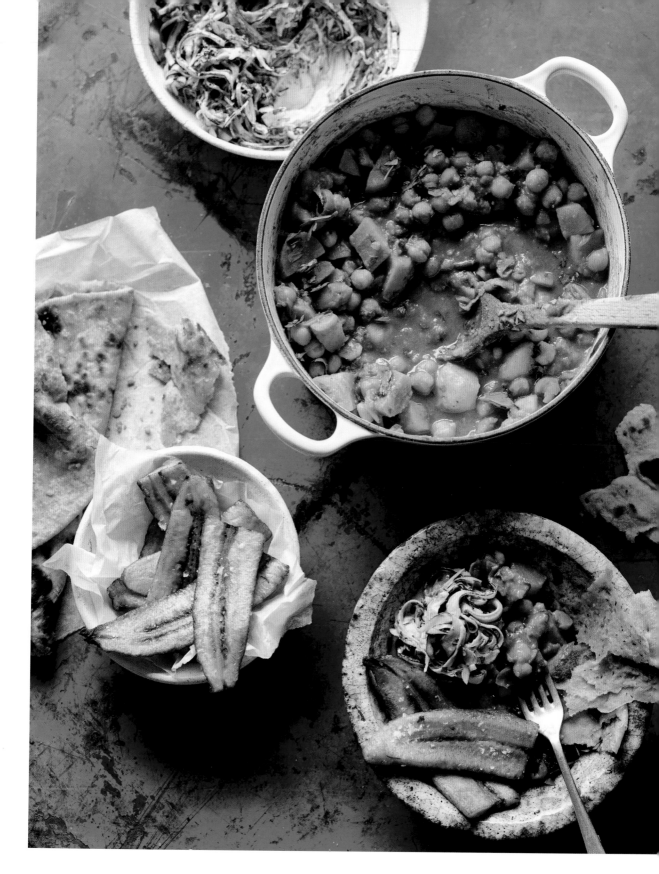

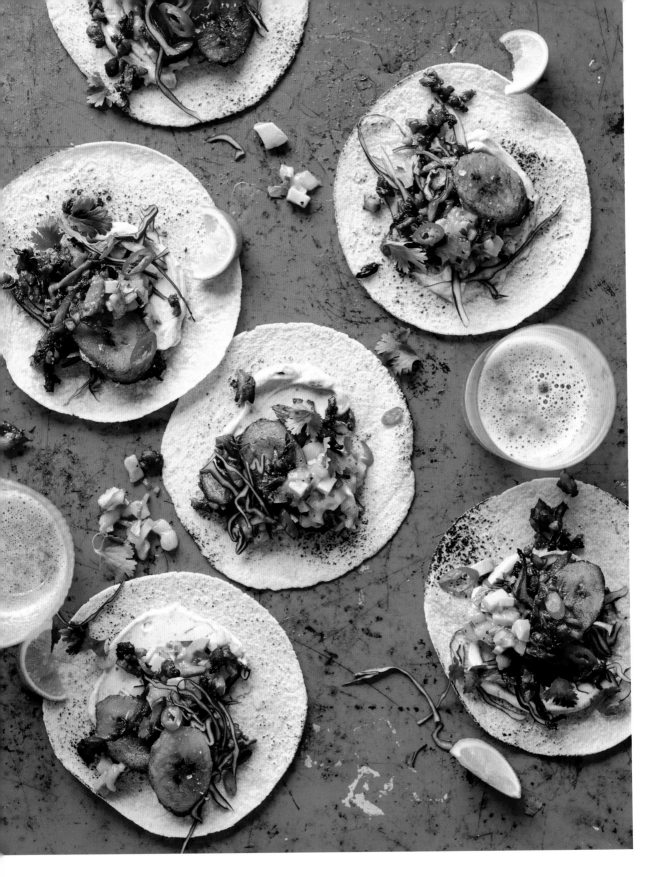

Dinner

Makes 8 tacos

8 small soft flour tortillas
½ head of red cabbage,
    finely sliced
1 quantity of Mango Avocado
    Salsa (see page 181)
1 quantity of Fried Plantains
    (see page 174)
1 lime, each cut into
    4 wedges
Handful of fresh coriander,
    finely chopped
2 spring onions,
    finely chopped
2 fresh red chillies, deseeded
    and finely sliced

**For the jerk
barbecue mushrooms**
500g oyster mushrooms,
    roughly chopped
1 tbsp olive oil
120ml Jerk Barbecue Sauce
    (see page 187)

For the jerk mayonnaise
90ml vegan mayonnaise
    (to make your own,
    see page 189 or 190)
1 tbsp dried jerk seasoning

Crispy Jerk Barbecue Tacos

A Caribbean twist on a classic Mexican taco. Oyster mushrooms are marinated in a sweet and spicy barbecue jerk sauce, roasted until crispy and then served in a tortilla with a cooling salsa, crunchy red cabbage, fresh lime juice, jerk mayonnaise and, of course, some fried plantains. These incredibly tasty tacos get me dancing every damn time!

Preheat the oven to 180°C fan.

In a bowl, mix together the oyster mushrooms with the olive oil and half the jerk barbecue sauce until the mushrooms are well coated.

Place the sauce-coated mushrooms on a baking tray and bake in the oven for 20 minutes. Remove the tray from the oven, toss the mushrooms, add the rest of the jerk barbecue sauce and then bake for another 20 minutes. Because of the sugar in the jerk sauce, keep an eye on the mushrooms to ensure they don't burn, reducing the heat if necessary.

Meanwhile, mix the mayonnaise with the jerk seasoning.

Fill each of the tortillas with some of the sliced red cabbage, mango avocado salsa, fried plantains, jerk mayonnaise and jerk barbecue mushrooms, sprinkle over some lime juice, coriander, spring onions and chillies and then fold up to serve.

BEENIE MAN (FEAT. MS THING) – 'DUDE'

Serves 4

2 aubergines, chopped
  into small chunks
2 courgettes, chopped
  into small chunks
2 red peppers, deseeded
  and chopped into
  small chunks
3 tbsp olive oil
2 red onions, diced
4 garlic cloves,
  finely chopped

Leaves from 2 thyme sprigs
2 × 400g tins
  of plum tomatoes
1 × 400g tin of chickpeas,
  drained and rinsed
1 tbsp balsamic vinegar
1 tbsp fresh lemon juice
Salt and black pepper
Handful of fresh coriander,
  roughly chopped,
  to garnish

Chickpea Ratatouille

A twist on a classic ratatouille with chickpeas for protein and extra fibre – and just because chickpeas are so amazing and versatile. I love to make the recipe in one big batch at the start of the week and have it over the next few days with a variety of different sides – sometimes brown rice and green veggies, sometimes potatoes – or even mixed in with pasta.

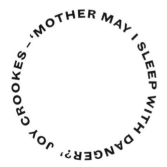

JOY CROOKES – 'MOTHER MAY I SLEEP WITH DANGER?'

Preheat the oven to 200°C fan.

Put the aubergines, courgettes and peppers on a baking tray, drizzle with 2 tablespoons of the olive oil and season with salt and pepper. Place in the oven to roast for 20 minutes, then remove from the oven, toss everything together and return to the oven to roast for another 10 minutes.

Meanwhile, pour the remaining olive oil into a large saucepan, add the onions and sauté over a medium heat for 4–5 minutes. Add the garlic and thyme, season with salt and pepper and cook for another 5–6 minutes, stirring frequently, until soft and browned.

Pour in the tinned tomatoes, then add the chickpeas, balsamic vinegar and lemon juice and season with salt and pepper. Mix everything together well, then cover the pan with a lid, bring to a simmer and cook on a low heat for about 20 minutes. Remove the lid, stir in the roasted vegetables and simmer for another 10 minutes until thickened. Taste and add more salt and pepper if needed.

Once cooked, remove from the heat and garnish with the coriander to serve.

Dinner

Serves 4

1 tbsp vegetable oil
5 shallots, diced
2 celery sticks,
    finely chopped
4 garlic cloves,
    finely chopped
1 rosemary sprig
3 fresh bay leaves
150ml vegan red wine
2 tbsp plain flour
500g all-purpose potatoes
    (such as Desiree),
    peeled and chopped
    into small chunks
4 carrots, peeled and chopped
    into small chunks

1 × 400g tin of
    chopped tomatoes
1 tbsp brown miso paste
500ml vegetable stock,
    plus more if needed
1 tsp vegan
    Worcestershire sauce
1 tbsp tomato purée
1 tsp vegan gravy
    browning (optional)
Salt and black pepper
Handful of fresh parsley,
    roughly chopped,
    to garnish

For the mushrooms

375g oyster mushrooms
2 tsp sweet smoked paprika
1 tbsp liquid smoke
    (optional)
2 tbsp soy sauce (or tamari
    sauce or coconut aminos)
1 tbsp maple syrup
1 tbsp vegetable oil

Beefless Stew with Oyster Mushrooms

One of my most popular recipes on YouTube is this warming hearty stew, packed with rich, savoury umami flavours. The oyster mushrooms give it a slightly chewy but soft texture (replacing the meat in a traditional beef stew). If you can't get hold of oyster mushrooms, you can use shiitake or Portobello, but I particularly love the texture of oyster mushrooms for this recipe.

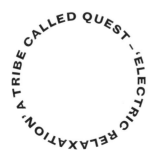

A TRIBE CALLED QUEST – 'ELECTRIC RELAXATION'

Place the vegetable oil in a large saucepan, add the shallots and celery and sauté over a medium heat for 4–5 minutes until softened. Add the garlic, rosemary sprig and bay leaves, season with salt and pepper and cook for 3–4 minutes, stirring frequently, until the garlic softens and the shallots and celery are lightly browned.

Pour in the red wine and bring to the boil, then reduce the heat and simmer until the liquid reduces by half.

Mix in the flour and add the potatoes and carrots. Add the tomatoes, miso paste and vegetable stock (adding more, if needed, to cover the vegetables in the pan), followed by the Worcestershire sauce, tomato purée and gravy browning (if using). Mix everything together well and cover the pan with a lid. Bring to the boil, then reduce the heat and leave to simmer for 15 minutes while you prepare the mushrooms.

In a bowl, mix the mushrooms in the paprika, liquid smoke (if using), soy sauce and maple syrup. Place the vegetable oil in a griddle pan (or a heavy-based frying pan) set over a medium heat and add the mushrooms in a single layer. Cook for 5–6 minutes, stirring occasionally, until lightly caramelised and crispy. (You may need to cook them in batches, depending on the size of your pan.)

Add the cooked mushrooms to the stew and simmer for another 15 minutes, uncovered, until the carrots and potatoes are tender and the sauce has thickened. Taste and add more salt and pepper if needed. Take off the heat, remove the rosemary and garnish with the parsley.

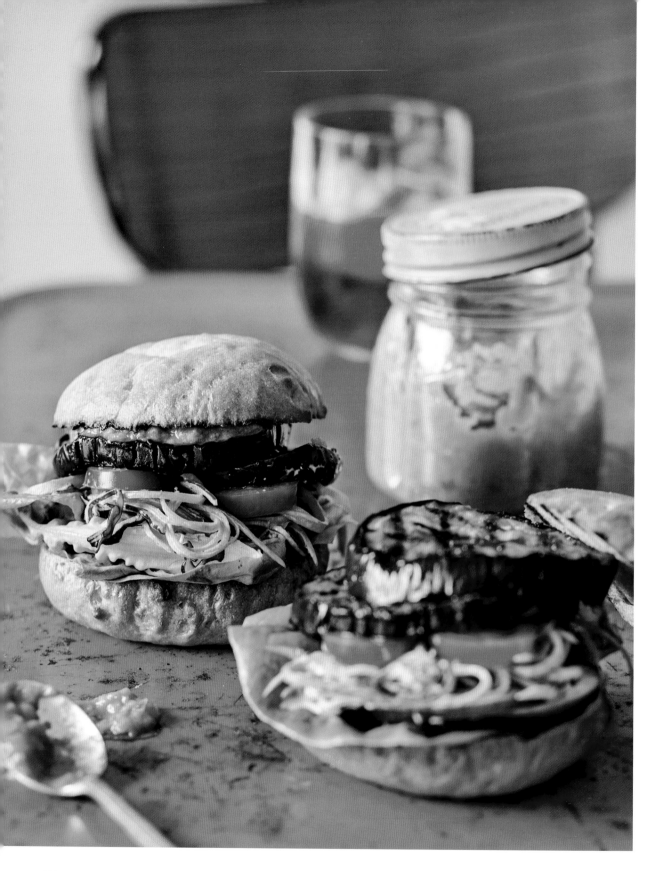

Dinner

Serves 4

1 tbsp vegetable oil
1 large wide aubergine, cut crossways into 1cm slices
60ml Jerk Marinade (see page 185)
4 vegan burger buns
1 quantity of Red Cabbage Slaw (see page 155)

2 tomatoes, sliced
1 red onion, finely sliced
Handful of fresh lettuce leaves
1 quantity of Mango Pineapple Ketchup (see page 188)
Salt and black pepper

Jerk Aubergine Burgers

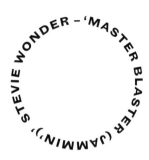

STEVIE WONDER – 'MASTER BLASTER (JAMMIN')'

Aubergines must be one of my favourite vegetables of all time and I love the texture of griddled aubergines in particular. Cooked in a spicy jerk marinade and served in a burger bun with red cabbage slaw, tomatoes, lettuce and mango pineapple ketchup, these burgers are so juicy and irresistible.

Place the oil in a griddle pan (or a heavy-based frying pan) set over a medium–high heat. Add the aubergine slices in a single layer, sprinkle with salt and pepper and cook for 5 minutes on each side until tender and lightly chargrilled. Brush with the jerk marinade, turn over and cook for 2 minutes, then brush the other side with the marinade and turn to cook for another 2 minutes.

Slice the burger buns in half. Add some red cabbage slaw to the lower half of each bun, followed by some tomato and red onion slices, griddled aubergines, lettuce leaves and mango pineapple ketchup. Sandwich together with the top half of each bun to serve.

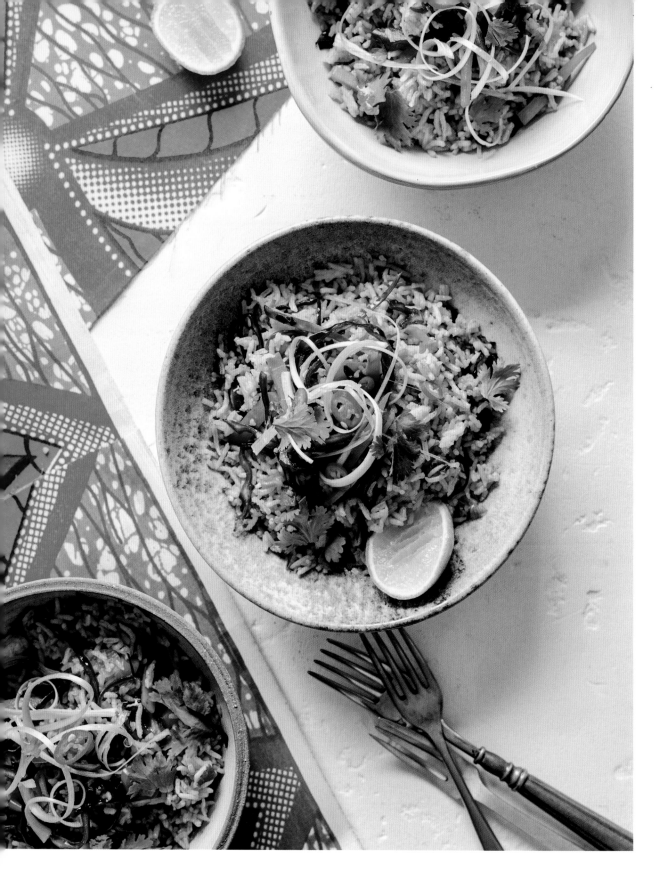

Dinner

Serves 4

400g basmati rice
2 tbsp coconut oil
3 shallots, finely chopped
6 garlic cloves,
    finely chopped
8 spring onions, chopped
2 carrots, peeled and
    finely sliced

½ white cabbage,
    thick ribs removed and
    leaves finely sliced
1 tbsp maple syrup
1 tbsp vegan fish sauce
    (to make your own,
    see page 193; optional)
2 tbsp soy sauce
    (or coconut aminos)
1 tbsp harissa paste
Salt and black pepper

To serve

2 fresh red chillies, deseeded
    and finely chopped
Handful of fresh coriander,
    roughly chopped
2 limes, each cut into
    4 wedges

Vegetable Coconut Fried Rice

This quick and simple fragrant fried rice dish is inspired by the Indonesian classic nasi goreng, which I ate nearly every day when I was on holiday in Bali a few years ago. For an extra hit of coconutty flavour, you could make it with the Coconut Rice on page 171. If you don't have vegan fish sauce, that's fine – just miss it out. This recipe is great for using any day-old rice and veg that you have in the fridge. Sometimes I vary between red and white cabbage, depending on what's calling me more.

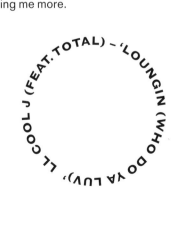

Rinse the rice thoroughly under the cold tap until the water runs clear, to remove any excess starch, then place the rice in a large saucepan with double the quantity of water and a good pinch of salt. Stir the rice in the water and then bring to the boil. Put a lid on top of the pan, reduce the heat to as low as possible and cook for 10 minutes, then take off the heat and leave, covered with the lid, for 5 minutes until the rice is tender and all the water has been absorbed. Remove the lid and fluff up the grains of rice with a fork.

Once cooked, set the rice aside to cool down completely. This recipe works best with day-old rice, so if time allows, run the cooked rice under the cold tap until cool, then drain and store in an airtight container in the fridge overnight or for a minimum of 3 hours.

Melt the coconut oil in a large frying pan or wok set over a medium heat. Add the shallots and cook for 4–5 minutes until they have softened and are lightly browned. Add 6 of the spring onions, followed by the carrots and cabbage, and cook for another 3 minutes, stirring occasionally.

Increase the heat to medium–high and add the maple syrup, vegan fish sauce (if using), soy sauce and harissa paste. Mix in well and then stir in the rice and season with salt and pepper. Stir-fry the mixture for about 5 minutes until the rice is piping hot, then remove from the heat.

Sprinkle with the remaining spring onions, the chopped chillies and coriander and serve with the lime wedges.

1–2 tbsp peanut oil

500g sweet potatoes, peeled and diced

1 × 400g tin of black-eyed peas, drained and rinsed

½ fresh red Scotch bonnet chilli, deseeded and kept whole (optional)

3 tbsp tomato purée

1 × 400g tin of chopped tomatoes

500ml vegetable stock

125g natural smooth peanut butter (to make your own, see page 240)

200g spinach, chopped

1 tbsp fresh lemon juice

Handful of fresh coriander, roughly chopped

2 spring onions, finely chopped

1 fresh red chilli, deseeded and finely sliced

Salt and black pepper

For the paste

2 onions, roughly chopped

5 garlic cloves, roughly chopped

Thumb-sized piece of fresh root ginger, peeled and roughly chopped

1 tsp paprika

2 tsp ground coriander

1 tsp ground turmeric

2 tsp ground cumin

1 tsp ground fenugreek

½–1 fresh red Scotch bonnet chilli (to taste), deseeded and roughly chopped

Pinch of salt

African Peanut Stew

My mum spent many summers in Sierra Leone, where her dad comes from, and this peanut stew was one of her favourite dishes. She usually had it with chicken, but when I made this plant-based version for her to try, she had the biggest smile on her face. This recipe is a definite winner in our house, perfect for when you want a really hearty and comforting dinner with a nice touch of spice to set your taste buds tingling. My favourite way to eat this is with plantains and coleslaw (see pages 174 and 155) or a light fresh salad.

Scotch bonnet chillies can be really hot depending on where they're from and how ripe they are. For a more gentle heat, you can place half a Scotch bonnet – deseeded but not cut up – into the stew to cook, then simply remove it before serving. This way the chilli flavour can infuse the stew but without adding too much heat. This is a great option if you are new to this quite fiery chilli pepper.

Place all the paste ingredients in a food processor and blitz into a coarse paste.

Heat 1 tablespoon of the peanut oil in a large, heavy-based saucepan or shallow frying pan. Add the paste and sauté over a medium–low heat for 10 minutes, stirring occasionally and adding a little more oil if the paste starts to stick to the pan.

Add the sweet potatoes, black-eyed peas, Scotch bonnet chilli (if using – see introduction) and tomato purée and mix to combine. Pour in the tinned tomatoes and vegetable stock, add the peanut butter, season with salt and pepper and stir in well. Cover the pan with a lid and bring to the boil, then reduce the heat and simmer for 25 minutes, stirring occasionally.

Remove from the heat and stir in the spinach, leaving it to wilt in the pan for 5 minutes. To finish, add the lemon juice, coriander, spring onions and sliced chillies and check the seasoning, adding more salt and pepper if needed.

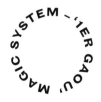

MAGIC SYSTEM – '1ER GAOU'

A classic you will hear all over Africa at weddings and other celebrations.

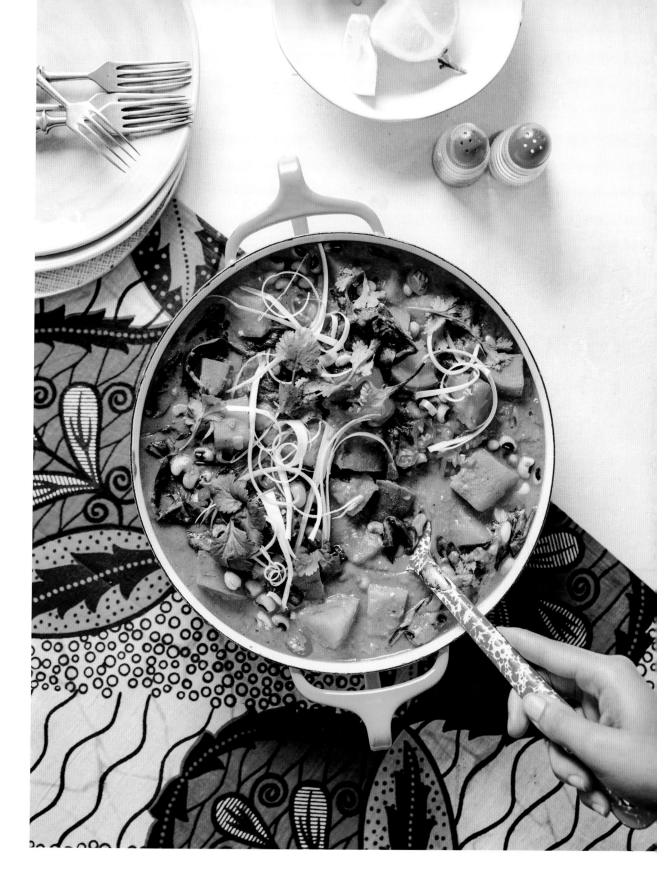

12 small soft flour tortillas
1 quantity of Guacamole
    (see page 180)
1 quantity of Cherry Tomato
    Salsa (see page 182)
Handful of lettuce leaves
Handful of fresh coriander,
    roughly chopped
2 limes, each cut into
    4 wedges

For the filling

1 tbsp vegetable oil
2 red onions, thinly sliced
2 red peppers,
    deseeded and sliced
2 yellow peppers,
    deseeded and sliced
4 garlic cloves,
    finely chopped
1 tbsp fajita seasoning
Salt and black pepper

Mexican Fajitas

When in need of a simple vibrant meal, I always turn to fajitas. Spicy peppers and onions with fresh-tasting guacamole, tomato salsa and crunchy lettuce all rolled up in a soft flour tortilla – so delicious! They're quick to make and are packed with some of my favourite flavours – great for when you've got friends over too, as they're hassle free. You could add black or refried beans for a more filling wrap or even chunks of your favourite vegan meat substitute.

Pour the oil into a large frying pan, add the onions and peppers, sprinkle with salt and pepper and sauté over a medium heat for 15 minutes, stirring occasionally, until softened and lightly browned. Add a splash of water if the onions and peppers start to catch.

Mix in the garlic and fajita seasoning and cook for another 5 minutes until the garlic has softened.

Then, make your wraps! Spread out each tortilla, add some of the pepper mixture, followed by a spoonful of guacamole and cherry tomato salsa and a few lettuce leaves, then sprinkle with the chopped coriander, add a squeeze of fresh lime juice and roll up to serve.

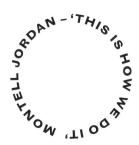

MONTELL JORDAN – 'THIS IS HOW WE DO IT'

Serves 4

For the spiced aubergines and chickpeas
2 large aubergines, chopped into 1cm cubes
5 tbsp olive oil
1 large onion, finely sliced
5 garlic cloves, finely chopped
1 tbsp ras el hanout
2 × 400g tins of chopped tomatoes
2 tbsp tomato purée
1 × 400g tin of chickpeas, drained and rinsed
Juice of ½ lemon
Handful of fresh parsley, roughly chopped
Salt and black pepper

For the green tahini dressing
240ml tahini
60ml water
1 tbsp maple syrup
1 tbsp extra-virgin olive oil
2 tbsp fresh lemon juice
Handful of fresh parsley, finely chopped
Handful of fresh coriander, finely chopped

To serve
Handful of rocket leaves
Handful of fresh parsley, roughly chopped
2 tbsp pumpkin seeds
2 lemons, each cut into 4 wedges
1 quantity of Sweet Potato Mash (see page 164)

Spiced Aubergines and Chickpeas

These aubergines are oven-roasted and mixed with chickpeas and tomatoes spiced with aromatic Moroccan ras el hanout. Served with a helping of delicious sweet potato mash and a drizzle of creamy tahini to bring it all together – a real treat for the taste buds! See photo on page 2.

Preheat the oven to 180°C fan.

Place the aubergines on a baking tray in a single layer – use more than one tray if necessary. Brush the aubergine chunks all over with 4 tablespoons of the olive oil, then sprinkle with salt and pepper. Place in the oven to roast for 25 minutes, tossing halfway through the cooking time, until tender and lightly browned.

In a deep saucepan, heat the remaining tablespoon of olive oil, add the onion and sauté over a medium heat for 10 minutes until soft and caramelised. Add the garlic and ras el hanout and sauté for another 3–4 minutes until the garlic is cooked.

Add the tinned tomatoes, tomato purée and chickpeas and mix to combine with the onion and garlic. Season with salt and pepper and cover the pan with a lid, then bring to a simmer and cook over a low heat for about 15 minutes.

Meanwhile, make the green tahini dressing. Place the tahini in a bowl with the water, maple syrup, olive oil and lemon juice and mix to combine, adding more water, if needed, for a runnier consistency. Mix in the herbs and season to taste with salt and pepper.

Add the roasted aubergines to the tomatoes and chickpeas and mix in well, then add the lemon juice, sprinkle over the parsley and remove from the heat. Transfer to a serving dish, drizzle the green tahini dressing over the spiced aubergines and chickpeas, top with the rocket, parsley and pumpkin seeds and serve with the lemon wedges and the sweet potato mash.

1 tbsp olive oil

2 red onions, finely sliced

2 red peppers, deseeded and sliced

1 yellow pepper, deseeded and sliced

1 tbsp maple syrup

1 tbsp vegetable oil

500g oyster mushrooms, roughly chopped

3–4 tbsp Jerk Marinade (see page 185), to taste

Handful of parsley, finely chopped

Handful of coriander, finely chopped

Salt

For the gravy

2 tbsp Jerk Marinade (see page 185)

120ml water

1 tbsp maple syrup

1 tbsp cornflour mixed with 1 tbsp water (optional)

To serve

1 quantity of Rice and Peas (see page 172)

1 quantity of Fried Plantains (see page 174)

½ quantity of Grilled Corn on the Cob with Garlic Chilli Marinade (see page 158)

1 quantity of Red Cabbage Slaw (see page 155)

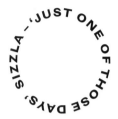

'JUST ONE OF THOSE DAYS,' SIZZLA –

Jerk Mushroom and Caramelised Onion Feast

During the Notting Hill Carnival in London there is always such hype around jerk chicken. I really wanted to share a recipe with my family and friends that avoided the chicken while still embracing those spicy jerk flavours, so I came up with this one. I tried it on a Caribbean chef and he loved it. Oyster mushrooms have such a great chewy, meat-like texture when griddled. Combined with caramelised onions, sweet peppers and a generous amount of jerk seasoning, plus a little jerk gravy, they're banging! I love this with a bit of coleslaw to cool it down, rice and peas and, of course, plantain.

Heat the olive oil in a large saucepan, add the onions and stir to coat in the oil, then sauté over a medium–low heat for 10 minutes, stirring occasionally. If the onions begin to dry out, add a splash of water.

Add the red and yellow peppers and sauté for another 10 minutes. If the mixture begins to dry out, add another splash of water if needed. Sprinkle with salt and add the maple syrup.

Meanwhile, place the vegetable oil in a griddle pan (or a heavy-based frying pan) set over a medium heat and add the mushrooms in a single layer. You may need to cook the mushrooms in batches, depending on the size of your pan. Once the mushrooms begin to brown, after 4–5 minutes, brush with the jerk marinade and continue to cook for 3–4 minutes until caramelised and charred.

Once the mushrooms are cooked, mix them in with the onions and peppers, then remove the pan from the heat and add the parsley and coriander.

To make the gravy, place the jerk marinade, water and maple syrup in a small saucepan. Bring to the boil, then reduce the heat and simmer for 5 minutes. For a thicker gravy, mix in the cornflour paste, then season to taste with salt and pour into a jug to serve.

Place the jerk mushroom and onion mixture in a serving dish and serve with the rice and peas, fried plantains, grilled corn on the cob, slaw and the jerk gravy.

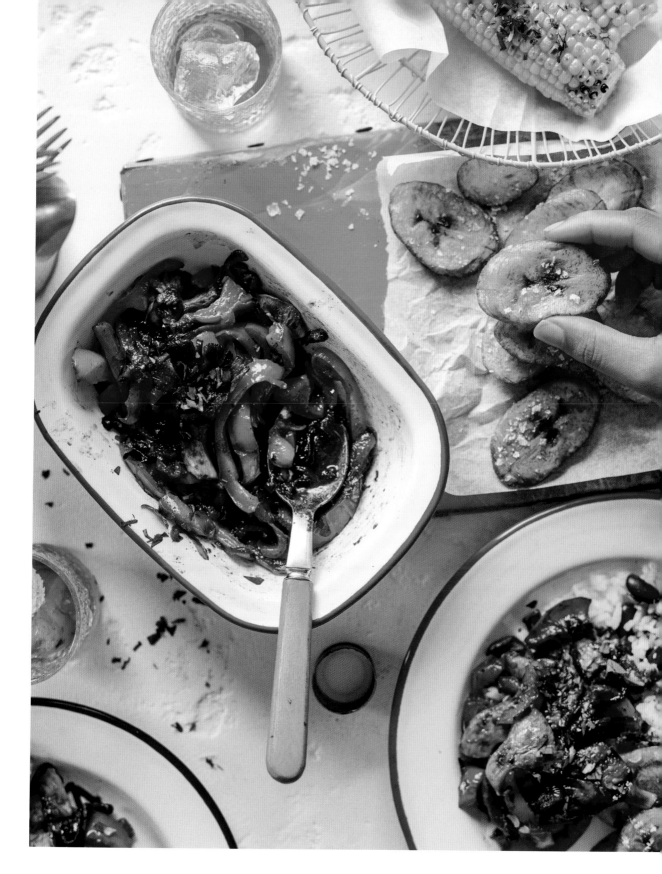

Serves 4

1 tbsp coconut oil

1 courgette, cut into chunks

1 head of broccoli, chopped
  into small florets

100g green beans, trimmed

400ml coconut milk

1 × 400g tin of chickpeas,
  drained and rinsed

100g mangetout

Handful of fresh
  Thai basil leaves

Salt and black pepper

**For the Thai green
curry paste**

4 garlic cloves,
  roughly chopped

3 shallots, roughly chopped

Thumb-sized piece of fresh
  root ginger, peeled and
  roughly chopped

2 lemongrass stalks, tough
  outer leaves removed,
  roughly chopped

4 green chillies, deseeded
  and roughly chopped

Stalks from a small handful
  of fresh coriander

1 tsp ground coriander

1 tsp ground cumin

1 tsp white pepper

1 tsp tamari sauce
  (or coconut aminos)

To serve

2 spring onions,
  roughly chopped

1 fresh red chilli, deseeded
  and finely chopped

Leaves from a small handful
  of fresh coriander,
  roughly chopped

2 limes, each cut into
  4 wedges

Thai Green Curry

The unique fragrant and delicate flavours of Thai cooking are reflected in this delicious Thai green curry paste, combined here with coconut milk, crunchy vegetables and chickpeas for a tasty vegan curry. This recipe is perfect for making a big batch and eating over the following 2–3 days; just serve it with brown rice for a wholesome meal. A more authentic way to prepare the paste is to use a pestle and mortar to break down the ingredients and get the flavours infusing together, but a food processor is very useful for making a quick paste if you are short of time or utensils.

Place all the ingredients for the Thai green curry paste in a food processor and pulse into a coarse paste. Alternatively, use a pestle and mortar to break down the ingredients.

Melt the coconut oil in a large pan over a medium heat, then add the courgettes, broccoli and green beans and sauté for 5 minutes. Add the Thai green curry paste to the pan, mix in until the vegetables are well coated and cook, stirring frequently, for another 5 minutes.

Pour in the coconut milk and add the chickpeas, then bring to the boil. Reduce the heat and cook for 3–4 minutes to heat through, seasoning to taste with salt and pepper. Add the mangetout and Thai basil and cook for another 3 minutes.

Remove from the heat and serve garnished with the spring onions, chilli, coriander and lime wedges.

Serves 4

1 tbsp coconut oil
2 onions, finely sliced
Thumb-sized piece of fresh
    root ginger, peeled and
    finely chopped
4 garlic cloves,
    finely chopped
1 tsp black mustard seeds
1 tsp cayenne pepper
1 tsp Madras curry powder

1 tsp ground coriander
1 tsp ground turmeric
1 × 400g tin of
    chopped tomatoes
200ml coconut milk
2 × 400g tins of chickpeas,
    drained and rinsed
Salt and black pepper
Large handful of fresh
    coriander, roughly
    chopped, to garnish

Curried Chickpeas

Quick and easy curried chickpeas bursting with flavour from the fragrant spices, tomatoes and coconut milk. Great with brown rice and a simple salad for a tasty and nourishing dinner.

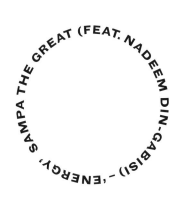

SAMPA THE GREAT (FEAT. NADEEM DIN-GABISI) – 'ENERGY,

Melt the coconut oil in a saucepan, add the onions and mix to coat thoroughly in the melted oil. Sauté over a medium heat for 7–10 minutes, stirring occasionally, until they are softened and start to caramelise.

Add the ginger and garlic, reduce the heat a little and sauté for 3–4 minutes until the garlic is almost translucent and has absorbed the oil. Now add all the spices and stir in well. If the onions look close to burning, stir in 1–2 tablespoons of water and mix well, taking care not to burn the spices either.

Pour in the tinned tomatoes, coconut milk and chickpeas and season with salt and pepper. Mix well, cover with a lid and bring to the boil, then reduce the heat and cook for 15 minutes on a low simmer.

Take off the lid and cook for a further 10 minutes to allow the sauce to reduce and thicken slightly. Then cover again and simmer on a low heat for another 20 minutes, stirring occasionally.

Remove from the heat and garnish with the chopped coriander to serve.

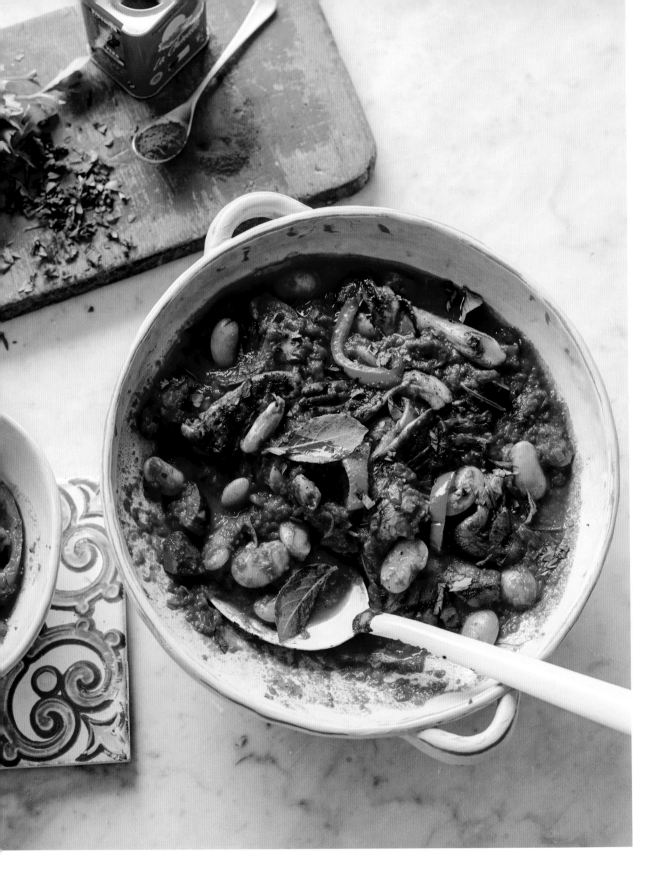

Dinner

Serves 4

1 tbsp olive oil
2 red onions, sliced
6 garlic cloves,
    finely chopped
1 courgette, roughly chopped
Leaves from 1 rosemary
    sprig, chopped
1 tbsp Spanish paprika
3 bay leaves
150ml vegan red wine
1 × 400g tin of
    chopped tomatoes
500ml vegetable stock
1 tbsp tomato purée

1 × 400g tin of butter beans,
    drained and rinsed
1 quantity of Roast Red
    Peppers (see page 154) or
    1 × 450g jar of roasted red
    peppers in oil, drained
Salt and black pepper
Handful of fresh parsley,
    roughly chopped,
    to garnish

For the mushrooms
375g oyster mushrooms
1 tbsp liquid smoke
    (optional)
2 tbsp soy sauce (or tamari
    sauce or coconut aminos)
2 tsp sweet smoked paprika
1 tbsp vegetable oil

Spanish Butter Bean Stew with Roast Peppers

A richly flavoured Spanish-inspired stew
with sweet roasted red peppers – super-hearty.
Perfect with rice, crispy potatoes or some bread
to soak up the juices.

Pour the olive oil into a large, deep saucepan or
flameproof casserole dish, add the onions and sauté
over a medium heat for 5–7 minutes until softened.
Add the garlic, courgette, rosemary, paprika and bay
leaves, season with salt and pepper and cook for
another 5 minutes.

Pour in the red wine and bring to the boil, then
reduce the heat and simmer until the wine reduces by
half. Tip in the tinned tomatoes and add the vegetable
stock, followed by the tomato purée. Mix well and cover
the pan with a lid, then bring back up to a simmer and
leave to cook over a medium–low heat.

Meanwhile, place the mushrooms in a bowl with the
liquid smoke (if using), soy sauce and smoked paprika,
season with salt and pepper and mix well until the
mushrooms are evenly coated.

Place the vegetable oil in a griddle pan (or a heavy-based
frying pan) over a gentle heat and add the soy-coated
mushrooms. Cook for 5–6 minutes, stirring occasionally,
until browned and any liquid has evaporated.

Add the mushrooms, butter beans and roast peppers
to the stew and cook for about 30 minutes in total, then
remove the lid and simmer until thickened. Taste, adding
more salt and pepper, if needed. Remove from the heat
and garnish with the parsley.

BUENA VISTA SOCIAL CLUB – 'CHAN CHAN'

4

SIDES, SAUCES AND DIPS

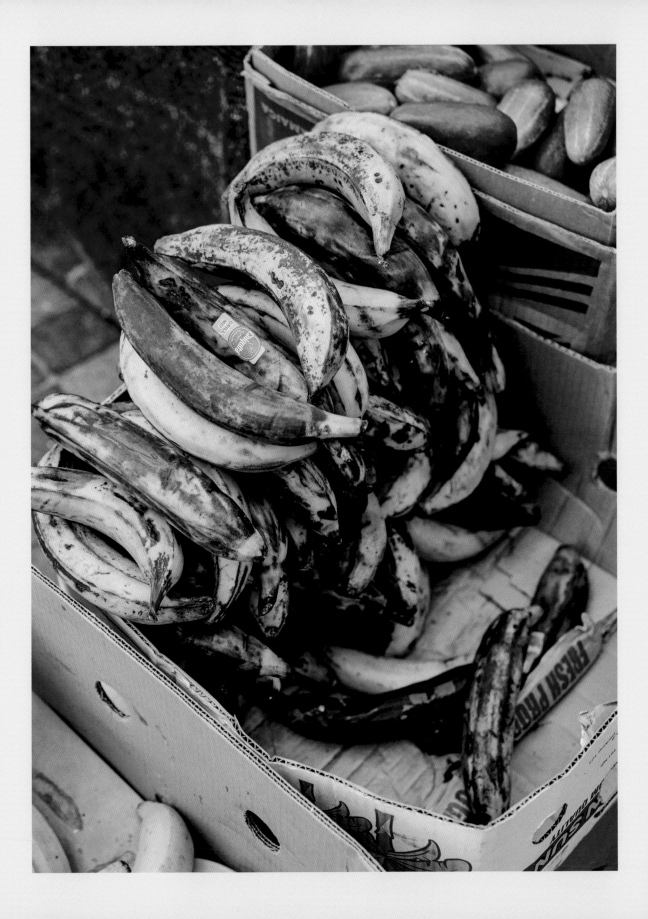

Sides, Sauces and Dips

These sides, sauces and dips are really amazing for adding extra texture and flavour to dishes in the dinner chapter, or you could even have a collection of the sides as one big feast!

If you're looking for quick and simple vegan mayo for your sandwiches, tropical ketchups for your plant-based burgers, tzatziki for your aubergine kebabs, hummus for – life in general, then this chapter has got you covered.

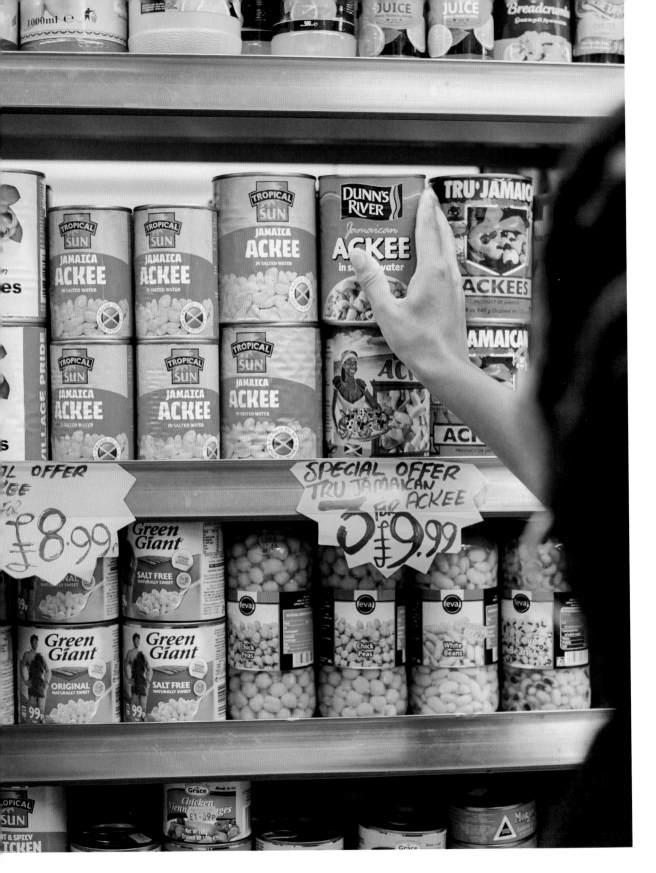

Sides, Sauces and Dips

Makes 6–8 dumplings

240g plain flour,
    plus extra for dusting
1 tbsp baking powder
1 tbsp soft brown sugar
¼ tsp salt
2 tbsp vegan butter,
    at room temperature
80ml water, at room
    temperature
Vegetable oil, for deep-frying

Caribbean Dumplings

Popular across the Caribbean, these are also known as Johnny cakes or bakes. These delicious fried dumplings are light and soft in the middle and golden and slightly crisp on the outside. Usually eaten for breakfast with traditional dishes such as ackee and saltfish (for my vegan version, see page 74), they can be served with many more dishes – especially when it comes to scooping up gravy. I used to love making these with my mum when I was growing up – they're so addictive!

LUCY PEARL – 'DANCE TONIGHT'

Sift the flour, baking powder, sugar and salt into a large bowl. Add the butter and rub it into the dry ingredients using your fingertips until the mixture resembles fine breadcrumbs, then mix in the water a little at a time to create a dough.

Tip the dough out onto a lightly floured worktop and knead to make it softer, then place back in the bowl, cover with a plate and leave in the fridge to rest for 20 minutes.

Remove the dough from the fridge and divide it into 6–8 pieces. On a lightly floured worktop, roll each piece into a ball.

Meanwhile, pour the oil into a deep heavy-based saucepan, ensuring that it is no more than two-thirds full, and heat the oil until it reaches 180°C on a food thermometer. Alternatively, drop in a cube of bread and, if it cooks in 30–40 seconds, the oil should be hot enough.

Using a slotted spoon, gently lower the dough balls into the hot oil to fry for 5–10 minutes, turning occasionally. Remove with the slotted spoon and place on kitchen paper or a clean tea towel to soak up any excess oil.

Once cooked, the dumplings should be light and fluffy and lightly browned on the outside.

Makes about 900g

2 × 400g tins of chickpeas, drained and rinsed

½ red onion, finely diced

110ml vegan mayonnaise (to make your own, see page 189 or 190)

2 tbsp nori flakes

1 tbsp fresh lemon juice

2 tbsp drained capers

2 tbsp soy sauce (or coconut aminos)

2 tbsp nutritional yeast

Salt and black pepper

Chuna

This is one of the first recipes I became obsessed with when I went vegan! It's remarkably similar to tuna mayonnaise but without the tuna. Soy sauce and capers are combined with nori flakes to create a sea-like saltiness that's evocative of seafood. A good source of protein, chickpeas also add texture. Use this to make amazing chuna salad sandwiches or as a classic filling for jacket potatoes (see page 76).

Place the chickpeas in a food processor or blender and pulse slightly. Alternatively, roughly mash the chickpeas using a fork or potato masher.

Tip the mashed chickpeas into a bowl, add the remaining ingredients and mix together well, seasoning to taste with salt and pepper.

If not using immediately, the chuna can be stored in the fridge in an airtight container for up to 2 days.

Makes about 30g

20g macadamia nuts

1 tbsp nutritional yeast

1 tbsp fresh white vegan
    breadcrumbs

½ tsp dried basil

½ tsp dried oregano

Herby Macadamia Crunch

A combination of nutritional yeast, creamy macadamia nuts, crunchy breadcrumbs and herbs – this is a super-tasty sprinkling for your pasta dishes. I love to use this as a Parmesan replacement and a tastier option than just adding nutritional yeast on top (although this is also great when you want a quick sprinkling of a savoury, slightly nutty flavour to your meals).

Place all the ingredients in a food processor and pulse into a coarse paste, or crush the nuts using a pestle and mortar and then mix with the other ingredients. Store in an airtight container in the fridge for 2–3 weeks.

Serves 4

60g brown miso paste
1 tbsp maple syrup
1 tsp harissa paste
1 tbsp fresh lemon juice
2 tbsp sesame oil
2 large aubergines,
   sliced widthways
1 tbsp white sesame seeds

1 tbsp pumpkin seeds
Handful of fresh parsley,
   roughly chopped
1 fresh red chilli, deseeded
   and finely chopped
2 spring onions, finely sliced

To serve
1 lemon, cut into 4 wedges
Handful of rocket leaves

Miso-glazed Aubergines with Rocket and Chilli

Quick and flavoursome oven-roasted aubergines marinated in a sweet and spicy miso sauce and served with fresh chillies and spring onions in a light salad. The perfect tasty quick snack or side dish for a big get-together! You can also cook these aubergines under the grill or in a griddle pan: just brush both sides with the marinade and cook for 10 minutes, turning once halfway through the cooking.

Preheat the oven to 200°C fan.

Place the miso paste and maple syrup in a bowl with the harissa paste, lemon juice and sesame oil and whisk until smooth.

Score a criss-cross pattern in the flesh of the aubergine slices on each side, then brush both sides with some of the miso mixture and set aside to marinate for 15 minutes.

Place the marinated aubergines on a baking tray and roast in the oven for 10 minutes, then remove from the oven, brush both sides with more marinade from the bowl and place back in the oven to cook for another 10 minutes or until tender and browned.

Meanwhile, toast the sesame seeds by sprinkling them into another baking tray and placing in the oven to cook for about 5 minutes, shaking the tray occasionally to ensure they don't burn, then set aside. You can toast the pumpkin seeds in the same way, if you like.

Transfer the roasted aubergines to a serving plate and sprinkle with the toasted sesame seeds, chopped parsley, chilli, spring onions and pumpkin seeds and serve with the lemon wedges and rocket leaves.

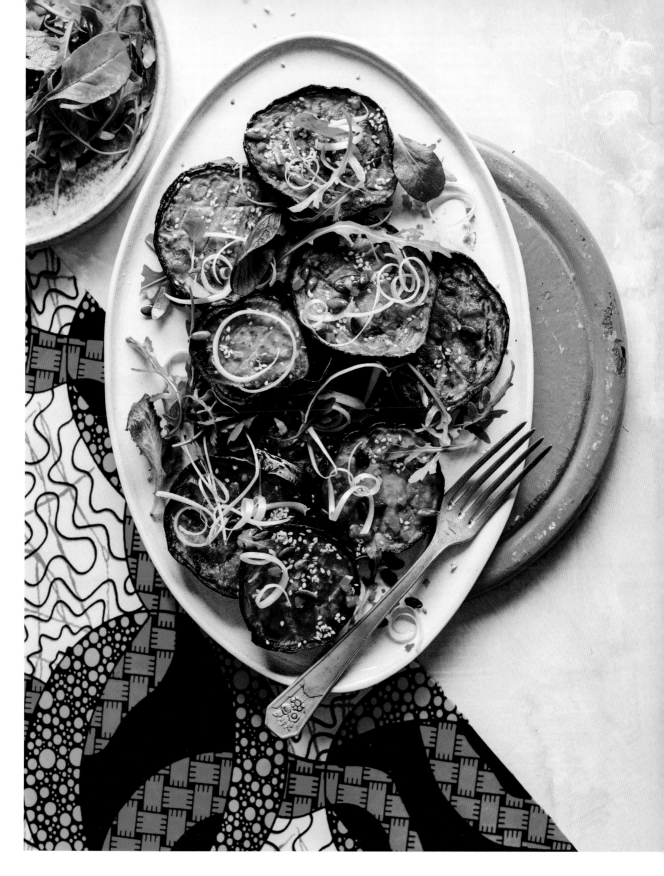

Serves 4

4–5 red peppers
2 tbsp olive oil,
    plus extra for greasing
Salt and black pepper
Handful of parsley,
    chopped, to garnish

Roast Red Peppers

Roasting red peppers is really simple: the heat of the oven brings out their natural sweetness, making these perfect for adding to salads, sandwiches or spreads.

Preheat the oven to 200°C fan and grease a baking sheet with olive oil or line with baking paper.

Place the peppers in the prepared baking tray and roast in the oven for about 25 minutes until the skins are wrinkled and lightly charred.

Transfer the cooked peppers to a bowl, cover with a plate and leave to cool for about 30 minutes.

When the peppers are cool, peel off the skins, then halve, deseed and slice into chunks or strips. Place the cooled pepper strips in a serving dish, drizzle with the olive oil and season to taste with salt and pepper, then garnish with the parsley to serve.

The pepper strips can be stored in the fridge in a sterilised jar (see page 175) with a lid for up to 5 days.

Serves 4

½ small red cabbage,
   shredded
½ small white cabbage,
   shredded
3 carrots, peeled and
   coarsely grated
4 spring onions,
   finely chopped

220ml vegan mayonnaise
   (to make your own,
   see page 189 or 190)
1 tbsp fresh lemon juice
Salt and black pepper
Handful of parsley, finely
   chopped, to garnish

Red
Cabbage
Slaw

Caribbean meals in my house always, always
went down with a side of plantain and a side of
coleslaw! This simple, fresh and crunchy coleslaw
is so perfect for cooling spicy dishes or for adding
taste and texture as part of a Caribbean Channa
feast (see page 124).

Place the cabbage, carrots and spring onions in a large
bowl. Add the mayonnaise and lemon juice and mix
together well, seasoning to taste with salt and pepper.

Transfer to a serving bowl and chill in the fridge for
30 minutes before serving garnished with the parsley.

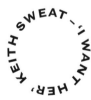

KEITH SWEAT – 'I WANT HER'

300g Tenderstem
 broccoli spears
1 tbsp olive oil
1 tbsp fresh lemon juice
Salt and black pepper

**For the lemon
tahini dressing**
50g tahini
3 tbsp fresh lemon juice
3 tbsp water
1 garlic clove, finely chopped
1 tbsp extra-virgin olive oil

Griddled Tenderstem Broccoli with Lemon Tahini Dressing

Heat up a griddle pan (or a heavy-based frying pan) over a high heat. In a bowl, toss the broccoli with the olive oil and lemon juice and season with salt and pepper.

Place the broccoli in the hot pan and chargrill for 8–10 minutes, turning occasionally, until the broccoli is lightly browned all over.

Meanwhile, mix together all the tahini dressing ingredients in a bowl and season to taste with salt and pepper. If the dressing is too thick, add a bit more water.

Place the chargrilled broccoli on a warmed serving plate and drizzle with the tahini dressing.

Transform your everyday broccoli with this delicious recipe – lightly crisp Tenderstem spears drizzled in a lemon tahini dressing. The perfect, extremely addictive side dish for the summer!

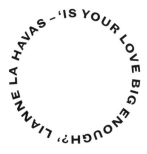

LIANNE LA HAVAS – 'IS YOUR LOVE BIG ENOUGH?'

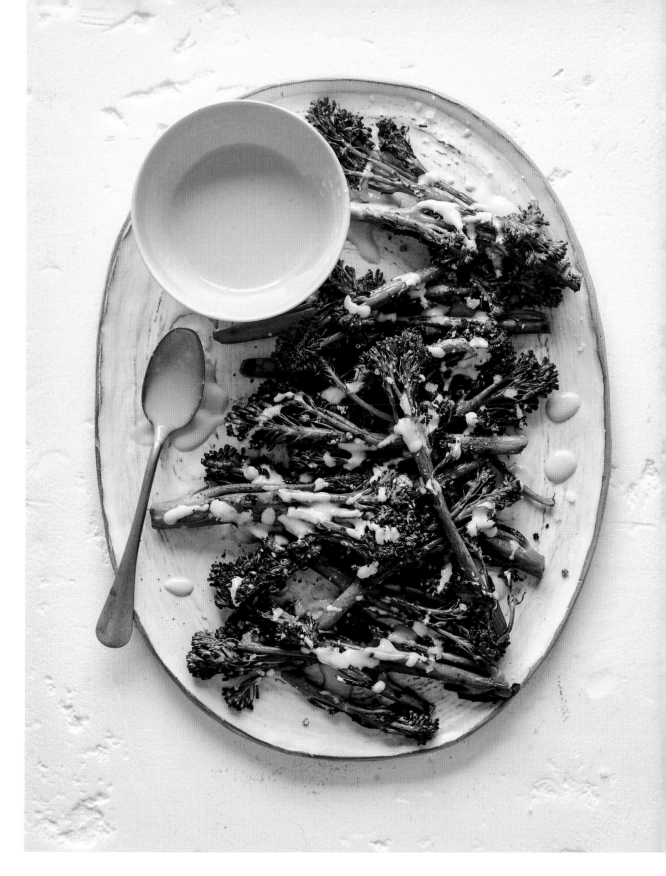

8 corn on the cob

**For the garlic
chilli marinade**
40g vegan butter
(or 2 tbsp vegetable oil)
Handful of coriander,
chopped, plus extra
to serve

Handful of parsley, chopped
1 fresh red chilli, deseeded
and finely chopped
1 garlic clove, finely chopped
Salt and black pepper

Grilled Corn on the Cob with Garlic Chilli Marinade

The ultimate classic summer side dish. Juicy, crunchy corn on the cob charred under the grill or on the barbecue for a smoky-sweet taste and seasoned with fresh herbs, garlic and chilli for extra punches of flavour. Perfect as part of a summer barbecue or even just to snack on.

Preheat the grill or barbecue to high.

In a bowl, combine the butter with the herbs, chilli and garlic. Season to taste with salt and pepper and then set aside.

Place the corn on the cob on the grill or barbecue and cook for about 5 minutes, turning occasionally. Use a pastry brush or a spoon to spread the marinade over the corn, ensuring that each piece is well covered, then cook for another 5 minutes, turning occasionally, until the corn is lightly charred all over. Sprinkle with extra coriander to serve.

Sides, Sauces and Dips

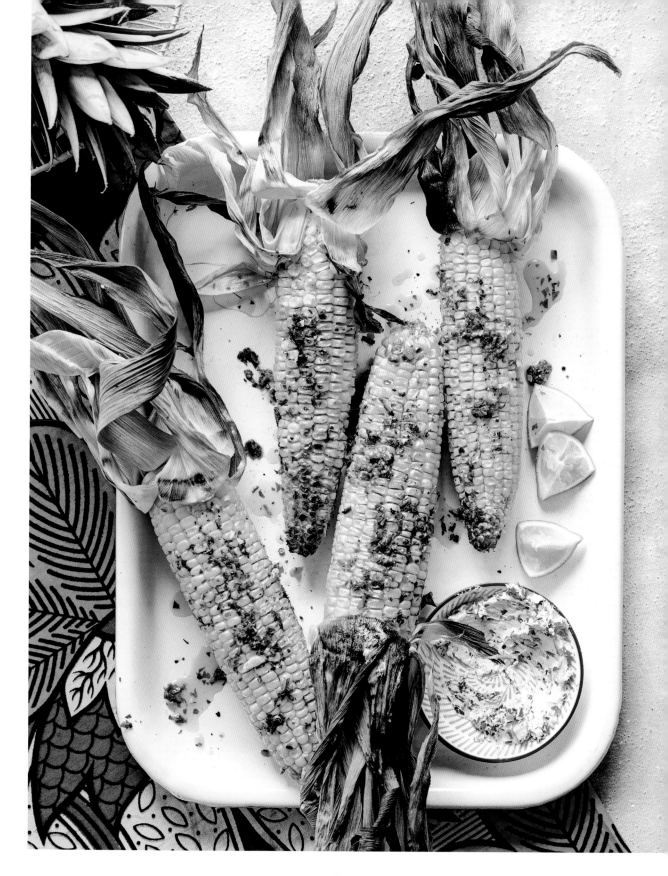

Serves 4

260g lettuce (such as
    butterhead), leaves
    roughly chopped
100g baby spinach
300g cherry tomatoes, halved
2 avocados, cut into cubes
2 spring onions, chopped
½ cucumber, chopped into
    small cubes

1 carrot, peeled and grated
Handful of broccoli sprouts
2 tbsp pumpkin seeds
Juice of ½ lemon
1 tbsp extra-virgin olive oil
Salt and black pepper
1 lemon, cut into
    4 wedges, to serve

My Go-to Salad

Place the salad leaves, vegetables, broccoli sprouts and pumpkin seeds in a serving bowl. Sprinkle over the lemon juice and olive oil, season to taste with salt and pepper and toss together well. Serve with the lemon wedges.

Toss all the ingredients together for this fresh and flavoursome salad and enjoy with summer dinners and lunches. I particularly love this salad with hummus, pitta and falafels or with griddled vegetables.

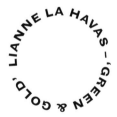

LIANNE LA HAVAS – 'GREEN & GOLD'

Serves 4

1 tbsp coconut oil
3 spring onions,
    finely chopped
3 garlic cloves,
    finely chopped
Leaves from 2 thyme sprigs
225g quinoa
240ml coconut milk

260ml water
1 × 240g tin of red kidney
    beans, drained and rinsed
½ fresh red Scotch
    bonnet chilli, deseeded
    (optional, for heat)
Salt and black pepper

Quinoa and Peas

A twist on the infamous Caribbean Rice and Peas (see page 172), swapping white rice with quinoa for the extra nutrients. This protein-packed combo works so deliciously well with coconut milk, creating a filling and slightly creamy side dish with a bit of a kick from the Scotch bonnet – perfect with vegetable stews and curries!

Melt the coconut oil in a large saucepan over a low heat, add the spring onions, garlic and thyme and cook for 4–5 minutes, stirring occasionally, until soft. Meanwhile, rinse the quinoa well under the cold tap.

Pour the coconut milk and water into the pan and stir in the kidney beans and Scotch bonnet (if using), then season with salt and pepper. Add the quinoa and bring to the boil, then reduce the heat and simmer for 10 minutes until all the liquid has been absorbed and the quinoa is soft and fluffy. Remove the Scotch bonnet before serving.

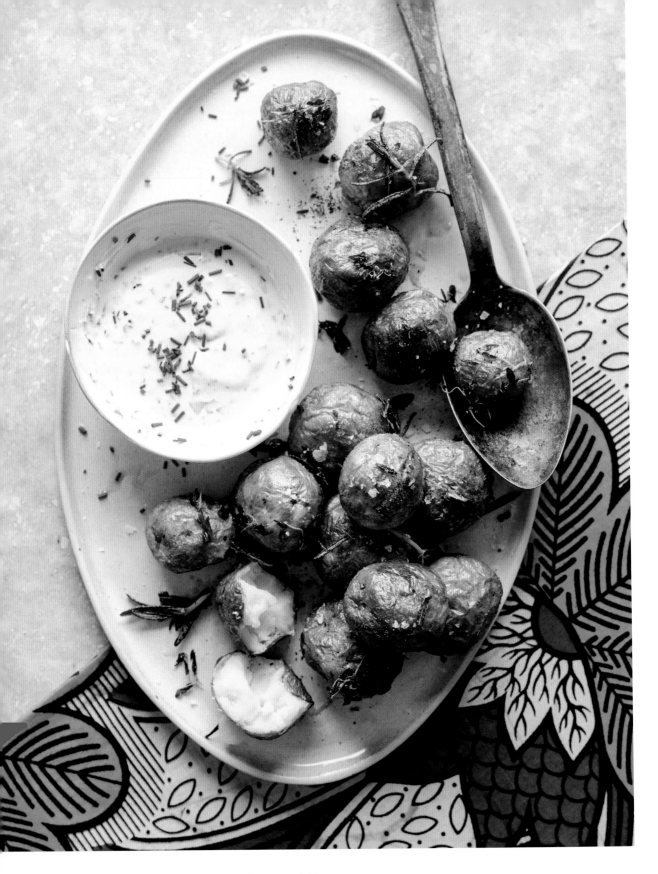

Sides, Sauces and Dips

Serves 4

2–3 tbsp olive oil

90g new potatoes (unpeeled)

Leaves from
2 rosemary sprigs

2 thyme sprigs

1 tbsp dried oregano

Salt and black pepper

For the aïoli

120ml Aquafaba Mayo
(see page 189)

1 tsp fresh lemon juice

2 garlic cloves,
finely chopped

Handful of fresh parsley,
finely chopped

1 tbsp finely snipped chives

Crispy New Potatoes with Herb Aïoli

Roasted with rosemary and thyme, these potatoes are beautifully crisp on the outside and soft and fluffy in the middle. Perfect for dunking in this flavoursome herb aïoli with its pungent garlic kick.

Preheat the oven to 200°C fan. Pour the olive oil into a roasting tin and place in the oven for 5 minutes to heat.

Rinse the potatoes well and pat dry with kitchen paper or a clean tea towel. Remove the roasting tin from the oven and add the potatoes and herbs, then season with salt and pepper and toss well in the hot oil.

Roast in the oven for 40–50 minutes, turning occasionally, until the potatoes are crisp and tender.

Meanwhile, place all the aïoli ingredients in a bowl and mix well to combine, seasoning to taste with salt and pepper.

Place the potatoes in a warmed serving dish and serve with the aïoli on the side.

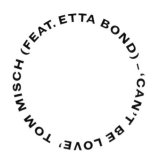

TOM MISCH (FEAT. ETTA BOND) – 'CAN'T BE LOVE'

Serves 4

3 large sweet potatoes,
  unpeeled and scrubbed
1 tsp ground cinnamon
½ tsp ground allspice
¼ tsp ground nutmeg
3 tbsp vegan butter
Salt and black pepper

Sweet Potato Mash

This is my favourite way to enjoy sweet potato mash – infused with a pinch of cinnamon, allspice and nutmeg.

Preheat the oven to 200°C fan.

Cut the potatoes in half lengthways and place them cut-side down on a baking sheet, then roast the sweet potatoes in the oven for about 25–30 minutes, or until cooked through.

Remove the sweet potatoes from the oven and allow to cool slightly, then slice in half and spoon the insides into a large bowl. Add the spices and butter and use a potato masher to mash to the desired consistency. Season to taste with salt and pepper.

Sides, Sauces and Dips

Makes 4 flatbreads

200g unsweetened
    coconut yoghurt
200g self-raising flour,
    plus extra for dusting
1 tsp ground turmeric
½ tsp baking powder
Pinch of salt

Optional extras
1 tsp dried herbs, ground
    cumin or chilli flakes
1 tbsp chopped fresh
    coriander

Coconut Turmeric Flatbreads

These really simple coconut flatbreads are so quick to make and are amazing for dipping into curries. You can spice them up a little and add some extra seasonings like cumin or coriander, or simply enjoy them as they are.

Place all the ingredients (including your chosen spice or herb, if using) in a large bowl and mix together into a rough dough. Tip out on to a lightly floured worktop and knead for 1 minute into a smooth dough, adding a little more flour if needed if the dough seems too wet. Split the dough into 4 equal-sized pieces and roughly flatten each piece into a round with your hands, or using a rolling pin, until about 2cm thick.

Heat a non-stick frying pan or griddle pan until hot and then add the flatbreads, one or two at a time. Cook for about 30 seconds on each side until lightly browned. Serve immediately while warm!

Makes 6–8 rotis

For the filling

¼–½ fresh red Scotch
 bonnet chilli (to taste),
 deseeded and finely
 chopped
110g dried yellow split peas
3 garlic cloves,
 roughly chopped
1 tsp ground cumin
½ tsp ground turmeric
Handful of coriander,
 roughly chopped
Salt (or pink Himalayan salt)
 and black pepper

For the dough

420g plain flour,
 plus extra for dusting
1½ tsp baking powder
¼ tsp ground turmeric
½ tsp salt
2 tbsp vegan butter
250–280ml warm water

120ml vegetable oil, for frying

Dhalpuri Rotis

Dhalpuri rotis are popular in the Caribbean, especially in Trinidad and Tobago where a lot of the cooking is influenced by eastern India. There are different types of roti – this is my favourite! Filled with a tasty mix of yellow split peas and a bold blend of spices, they're then cooked in a hot pan on the hob. Rotis are usually torn into pieces and used to scoop up all the delicious juices of stews, soups and curries or they are used to make wraps. Mastering the art of making these highly addictive flatbreads can take some practice but they are well worth perfecting!

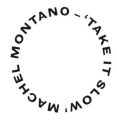

Place all the filling ingredients in a food processor and pulse until roughly broken down but not puréed. Season to taste with salt and pepper.

Sift the flour, baking powder, turmeric and salt into a large bowl, then rub the butter into the flour using your fingertips until the mixture resembles fine breadcrumbs. Slowly mix in the 250ml of the warm water to create a dough, adding the rest if the dough seems too stiff.

Knead the dough for 10 minutes on a lightly floured worktop until it is elastic and smooth, then cover with a clean tea towel and leave to rest for 30 minutes. Divide into 6–8 pieces and roll each piece into a ball.

With a rolling pin, on a lightly floured worktop, roll out each dough ball to a disc about 5mm thick, then place 2–3 tablespoons of the split pea mixture in the middle. Lift up the edges of the dough to enclose the mixture, pinching them together to seal the opening and smoothing the dough to ensure the filling doesn't leak.

Carefully roll each dough ball into a disc about 3mm thick, dusting the worktop with extra flour to help the roti stay together as you roll it out.

Brush a large frying pan or griddle pan with some of the vegetable oil and set over a high heat. Cook the rotis one at time for roughly 3 minutes on each side until lightly browned, brushing the pan with more of the oil as you cook each roti. Drain on kitchen paper or a clean tea towel to remove the excess oil and then serve. These are best eaten on the same day.

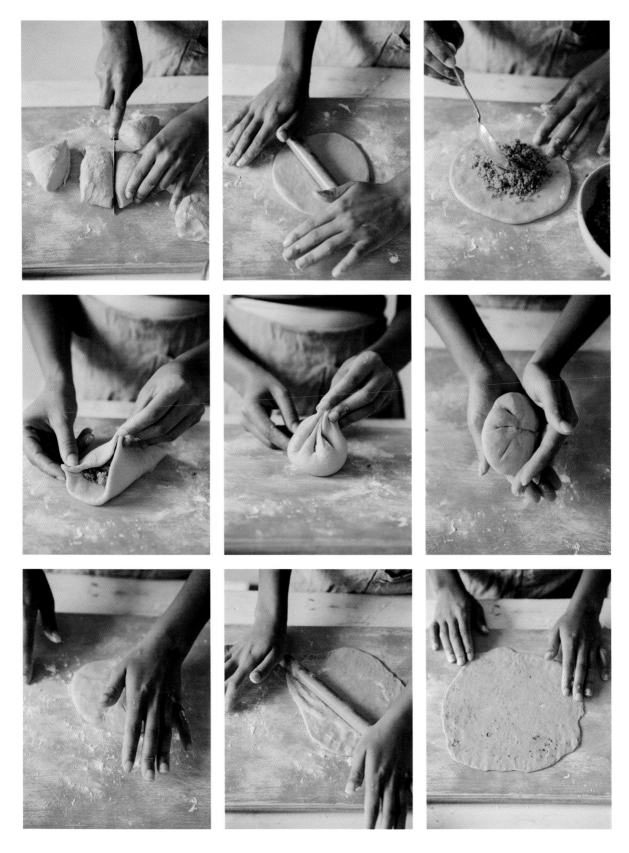

360g basmati rice

1 tbsp coconut oil

4 garlic cloves, finely chopped

200g green beans, trimmed

2 red peppers, halved, deseeded and cut lengthways into strips

2 fresh red chillies, deseeded and finely chopped, plus extra to serve

200g Tenderstem broccoli spears, thicker stems sliced

240ml Peanut Sauce (see page 192)

Juice of ½ lime

Salt and black pepper

To serve

1 lime, cut into 4 wedges

4 spring onions, chopped

Handful of fresh coriander, finely chopped

Peanut Fried Rice

Twist up your regular fried rice with an intensely satisfying peanut sauce. A delicious way to pack in your veggies, especially when using up bits and pieces in the fridge for a simple and filling meal. This recipe works best with day-old rice for a better texture, but it can also be made with fresh rice; just make sure the rice isn't overcooked or it will be too soft. You could also substitute the rice with noodles for a peanut noodle stir-fry.

Rinse the rice thoroughly under the cold tap until the water runs clear, to remove any excess starch, then place the rice in a saucepan with double the amount of water and a good pinch of salt. Stir the rice in the water and then bring to the boil. Put a lid on top of the pan, reduce the heat to as low as possible and cook for 10 minutes, then take off the heat and leave, covered with the lid, for 5 minutes until the rice is tender and all the water has been absorbed. Remove the lid and fluff up the grains of rice with a fork.

Once cooked, set the rice aside to cool down completely. This recipe works best with day-old rice, so if time allows, run the cooked rice under the cold tap until cool, then drain and store in an airtight container in the fridge overnight or for a minimum of 3 hours.

Heat a large frying pan or wok over a high heat, then add the coconut oil. When the oil has melted, add the garlic, green beans, red peppers, chillies and broccoli and cook for 5 minutes stirring frequently.

Add the cooked rice and stir-fry for about 5 minutes until the rice is hot, then add the peanut sauce, mixing it in well, and stir-fry for 2 minutes. Remove from the heat and add the lime juice.

Divide between plates and serve with the lime wedges and with the spring onions, chillies and coriander scattered over.

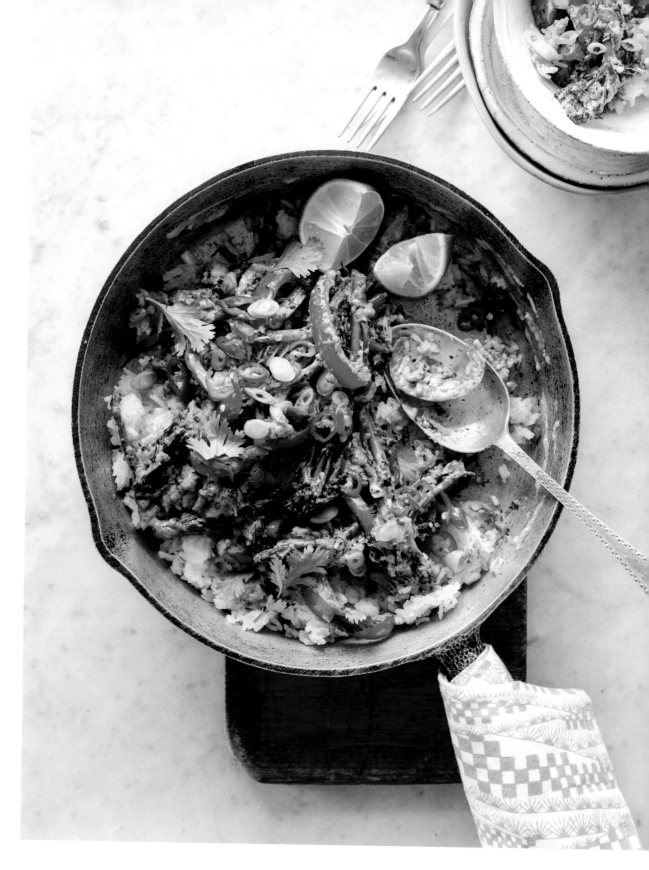

Serves 4

2 tbsp vegetable oil
2 red onions,
 roughly chopped
2 red peppers, deseeded
 and roughly chopped
4 garlic cloves,
 roughly chopped
1 tsp chopped fresh
 root ginger
½–1 fresh red Scotch bonnet
 chilli, deseeded and
 roughly chopped

2 tsp curry powder
Leaves from 2 thyme sprigs
2 large tomatoes,
 roughly chopped
4 tbsp tomato purée
500ml vegetable stock
300g basmati rice
3 bay leaves
Salt

Jollof Rice

Jollof rice is a true classic. Recipes vary across West Africa but the general concept is to cook the rice in a mixture of spices, herbs, vegetables and tomatoes all in one pot for the rice to soak up all the delicious flavours. In my house, it's usually accompanied with a side of plantain, slaw (see pages 174 and 155) and stewed beans or a vegetable dish. The debates we had in school about the merits of jollof versus Rice and Peas (see page 172) were never-ending, but being both African and Caribbean, I truly love them both! Use half a deseeded Scotch bonnet for a medium to low heat and a whole deseeded Scotch bonnet for medium to high heat; I like to use a whole pepper.

Place the vegetable oil in a large deep saucepan (which has a lid) over a medium heat, add the onions and cook for 5 minutes until they begin to soften. Add the red peppers, garlic, ginger, Scotch bonnet, curry powder, thyme leaves and sauté over a medium heat, stirring occasionally, for 10 minutes.

Stir in the chopped tomatoes, tomato purée and vegetable stock, mix well and simmer for 2 minutes.

Transfer the mixture to a food processor and blitz into a smooth sauce (put the pan to one side).

Measure out 600ml of the sauce (you can freeze any left over and simply use it in the same 2:1 ratio of sauce to rice).

Meanwhile, rinse the rice thoroughly under the cold tap until the water runs clear, to remove any excess starch. Then tip the rice into the pan you'd been using followed by the 600ml of sauce and mix well. Add the bay leaves, season with salt and bring to a boil. Reduce the heat to its lowest setting (if the heat is too high you risk burning the rice at the bottom of the pan), cover the pan with a lid and cook for 20 minutes.

Remove the lid and give the rice a stir, then put the lid back on top and cook at a very low heat for another 10 minutes or until the rice is tender and all the liquid has been absorbed.

Serves 4

1 tbsp coconut oil

5 garlic cloves,
    finely chopped

500g basmati rice

400ml coconut milk

400ml water

Salt

Coconut Rice

I became obsessed with coconut rice from my time travelling around Colombia, to the point that I don't really enjoy plain white rice as much any more. It has to be either coconut rice, Jollof Rice (see opposite) or Rice and Peas (see page 172)! This is my very simple method of making coconut rice inspired by my time travelling, made with a touch of garlic, the coconut milk imparting a sweet creaminess and nuttiness. It goes so well with curries and black bean stews such as Vegetable Chilli (see page 106) or incorporated into fried rice dishes. Why not serve it with a side of plantain too (see page 174)?

In a large deep pan, melt the coconut oil and then sauté the garlic over a low heat for 3–4 minutes until softened.

Meanwhile, rinse the rice thoroughly under the cold tap until the water runs clear, to remove any excess starch.

Pour the coconut milk and water into the pan, followed by the rice. Mix well to combine, season with salt and cover with a lid. Bring to the boil, then reduce the heat to medium–low and cook for 10 minutes or until the rice is tender and all the liquid has been absorbed. Remove the lid, take the pan off the hob and fluff up the rice with a fork.

1 tbsp coconut oil
2 spring onions, finely sliced
3 garlic cloves
Leaves from 2 thyme sprigs
400g basmati rice

400ml coconut milk
480ml water
2 × 400g tins of kidney beans,
    drained and rinsed
Salt and black pepper

Rice and Peas

A staple side dish across the Caribbean that goes with almost anything. The rice is cooked in coconut milk, and absorbs the creamy texture and slight nuttiness from the coconut as well as all the flavours from the spring onions, garlic and thyme. You can also substitute the kidney beans with pigeon (or gungo) peas, which some people prefer – I love both!

In a large deep pan, melt the coconut oil and sauté the spring onions, garlic and thyme over a medium heat for 5 minutes until softened. Meanwhile, rinse the rice thoroughly under the cold tap until the water runs clear, to remove any excess starch.

Tip the rice into the pan, followed by the coconut milk and water, and season with salt and pepper. Add the kidney beans, cover with a lid and bring to the boil, then reduce the heat to low and cook for 10 minutes or until the rice is tender and all the liquid has been absorbed. Remove the lid, take the pan off the hob and fluff up the rice with a fork.

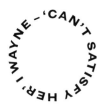

WAYNE - 'CAN'T SATISFY HER', I

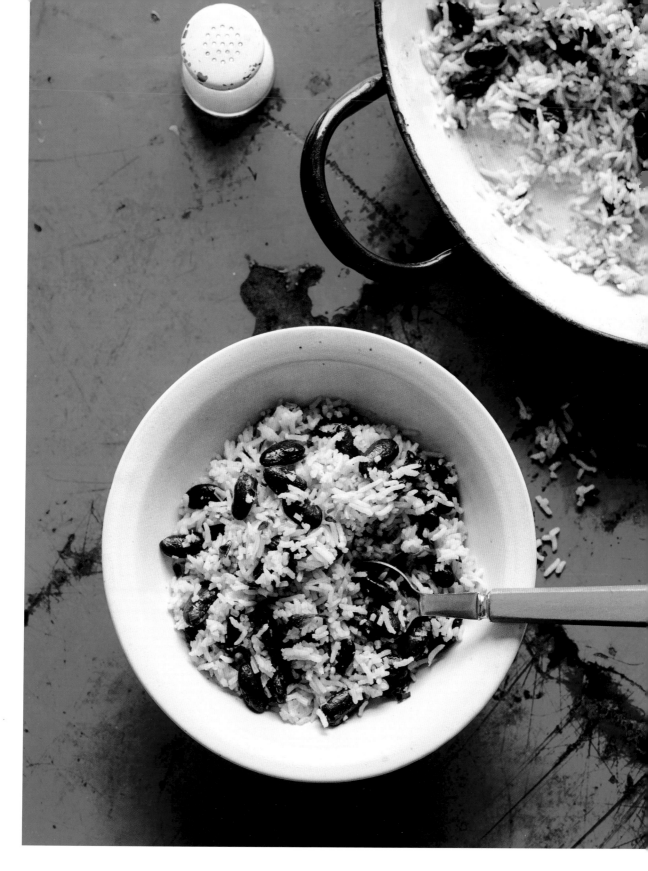

2 ripe plantains
2 tbsp vegetable oil
Salt

2 ripe plantains

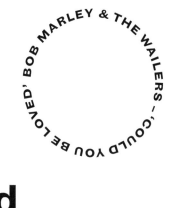

Fried Plantains

Baked Plantains

My love for fried plantains is a forever of love – probably one of my top five things to eat in the world. The darker the plantain, the riper and sweeter they are and less starchy. I love picking up black and yellow ones. Fried in vegetable oil, they caramelise and lightly crisp up on the outside. Sprinkle with a bit of sea salt before serving and you won't be able to stop snacking on them. You can deep-fry them in a large amount of oil, but I don't find that essential to achieve banging fried plantain.

An alternative to frying plantains in vegetable oil is to bake them. Choose ripe ones for sweetness, pop them in the oven to cook for 25 minutes and they come out so well – sweet, hot and delicious!

Preheat the oven to 180°C fan.

Place the plantains in their skins on a baking tray and roast in the oven for 25 minutes. Remove from the oven, then split the skins and remove the cooked plantains to serve.

Cut both ends off each plantain, then use a sharp knife to cut a shallow slit down the length of the plantain and remove the skin. Slice each plantain into thick pieces on the diagonal.

Heat the vegetable oil in a large frying pan over a medium–high heat. Add the plantain pieces and fry on each side for about 5 minutes until they are soft and golden brown all over. Sprinkle with salt before serving.

Sides, Sauces and Dips

Serves 4

12 large ripe tomatoes,
   halved
Olive oil, for drizzling
2 tbsp drained capers
Salt and black pepper

Slow-roast
Tomatoes

Perfect for adding to a sandwich, pasta or any salad. You can make this with smaller tomatoes or cherry tomatoes if you prefer – just halve the cooking time.

Preheat the oven to 140°C fan and line two baking sheets with baking paper.

Lay the tomatoes on the prepared baking trays, cut-side up, and drizzle a little olive oil over each tomato, then sprinkle them evenly with salt and pepper. Roast in the oven for 2 hours until tender and beginning to dry out.

Sprinkle the capers on to the baking sheets and return to the oven for a further ¾–1 hour or until the tomatoes are no longer wet and have shrunk slightly.

After cooling, the roast tomatoes can be stored in a sterilised jar (see below), covered with a layer of olive oil before sealing with a lid, and kept in the fridge for up to a week.

STERILISING JARS

To sterilise a jar and its lid, first wash in warm, soapy water, rinse well and then place on a baking tray in the oven, preheated to 120°C fan, and leave to dry for 10–15 minutes. Alternatively, put them through a hot dishwasher cycle and use immediately.

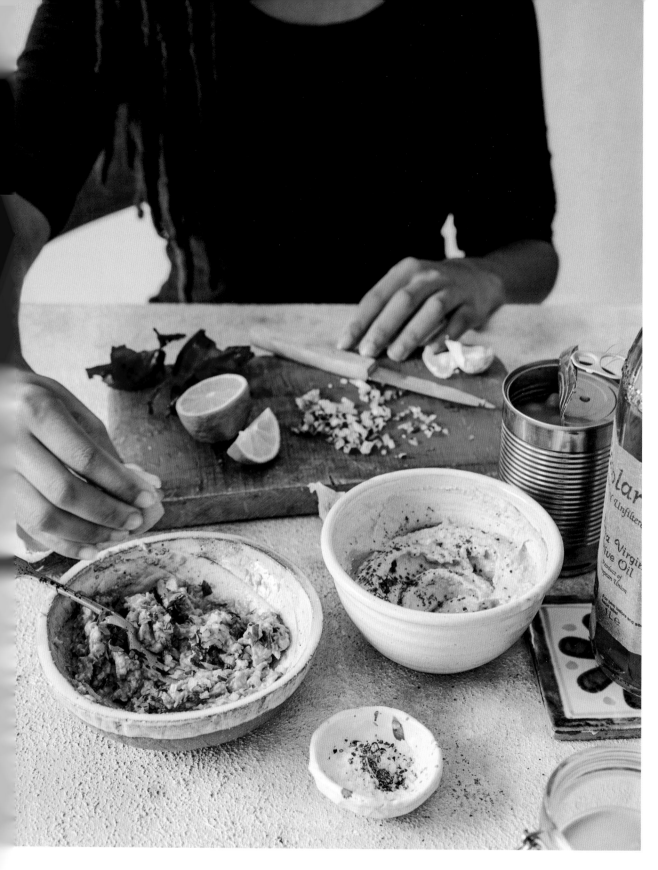

Sides, Sauces and Dips

Serves 4

2 × 400g tins of chickpeas,
  drained and rinsed
4 ice cubes
60ml extra-virgin olive oil,
  plus extra for drizzling
2–3 tbsp fresh lemon juice
  (to taste)
3–4 garlic cloves (to taste),
  roughly chopped
60g light tahini
Salt and black pepper

To serve

1 tsp paprika, ground
  sumac or ground cumin
  (optional)
1 tbsp finely chopped parsley

Hummus

This smooth, rich creamy hummus is high
in both protein and fibre, making it a nutritious
as well as delicious snack. Enjoy with a side of
warm flatbreads or pitta, add to sandwiches
or use as a dip – it's so versatile. I always have
hummus to hand in the house for those moments
of desperation or for when coming home after a
long night and needing a quick snack. Hummus
and wholemeal pitta bread every time!

Place the chickpeas in a food processor with the ice
cubes, olive oil, lemon juice, garlic and tahini, and blend
to a creamy purée. Season to taste with salt and pepper
and, if not serving immediately, store in the fridge in an
airtight container for up to 4 days.

To serve, transfer to a serving bowl, drizzle over some
extra olive oil and sprinkle with the paprika or other
spices (if using) and the parsley.

Makes about 300g

40g raw cashew nuts

280g extra-firm tofu, drained
and cut into chunks

2 tbsp coconut oil (optional)

1 tbsp nutritional yeast

2–3 tbsp fresh lemon juice
(to taste)

1 tsp garlic granules

Handful of fresh chives,
finely snipped

Salt and black pepper

Chive Tofu Spread

Made with tofu and cashews and mixed with fresh chives, this thick and creamy spread goes so well with crackers or on a bagel (see page 59). The coconut oil helps to keep the spread firm, but if you don't like the taste, you can just leave it out. See photo on page 52.

Cover the cashew nuts with water and leave to soak for 2 hours, then drain.

Gently press the drained tofu to remove as much moisture as possible, then place in a food processor with the drained cashews and all the other ingredients except for the chives. Blend until smooth, seasoning to taste with salt and pepper. Transfer to a bowl, fold in the chives and serve.

The spread can be stored in the fridge in an airtight container for up to 3 days.

Makes about 600g

300g raw cashew nuts
240ml water
2 garlic cloves,
    finely chopped
2 tbsp nutritional yeast
1–3 tbsp fresh lemon juice
    (to taste)
Handful of fresh basil leaves,
    finely chopped
Salt and black pepper

Basil Cashew Spread

Cashew nuts are fantastic for creating smooth and creamy sauces and spreads. This incredibly simple spread mixed with fresh basil makes a deliciously creamy dip and goes so well on a slice of toast or in a sandwich.

Cover the cashews with water and leave to soak for 2 hours, then drain.

Place the cashews in a food processor with the water, garlic, nutritional yeast and 1 tablespoon of the lemon juice. Season with salt and pepper and blitz until smooth.

Taste for seasoning, adding more salt and pepper or lemon juice, if needed. For a smoother, looser spread, you can add more water, 1 tablespoon at a time, until you reach the desired consistency.

Transfer the spread to a bowl and fold in the basil. The spread can be stored in the fridge in an airtight container for up to 3 days.

Serves 4

½ cucumber, grated
3 garlic cloves,
    finely chopped
3 tbsp finely chopped dill
1 tbsp fresh lemon juice
1 tsp finely chopped
    mint leaves
490g unsweetened
    coconut yoghurt
Salt and black pepper

Serves 4

2 ripe avocados
½ red onion, diced
1 tbsp fresh lime juice
Handful of fresh coriander
Salt and black pepper

Tzatziki

Guacamole

This delicious Greek-inspired dip is so fresh and simple, made with coconut yoghurt, garlic, fresh cucumber and lemon juice. I love this dip with the aubergine kebabs on page 102 or it's the perfect accompaniment to spiced grilled vegetables and pitta breads.

Such a fresh-tasting quick dish, made with minimal ingredients, guacamole is an absolute staple. When serving it as part of a big feast, it's always the first to go. See photo on page 176.

To make the tzatziki combine all the ingredients in a bowl, adding salt and pepper to taste.

Slice each avocado in half and remove the stone. Then, using a spoon, scoop out the avocado flesh from the skin and into a bowl. Use a fork to mash the avocado into the desired consistency, then stir in the remaining ingredients and season with salt and pepper to taste.

If not serving immediately, the guacamole can be kept in the fridge in an airtight container for up to 1 day before the avocado starts to go brown.

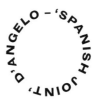

Serves 4

1 mango, finely diced
1 avocado, finely diced
½ red onion, finely chopped
1 red chilli, deseeded and
    finely chopped
2 tbsp extra-virgin olive oil
1 tbsp fresh lime juice
Handful of fresh coriander,
    finely chopped
Salt and black pepper

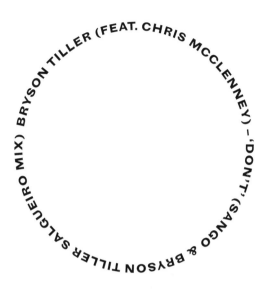

BRYSON TILLER (FEAT. CHRIS MCCLENNEY) – 'DON'T' (SANGO & BRYSON TILLER SALGUEIRO MIX)

Mango Avocado Salsa

Bursting with flavour from the sweet mango, diced avocado, fresh lime juice, chilli and coriander, this is a refreshingly sweet and slightly spicy side. The perfect accompaniment to summer dishes, for scooping up with tortilla chips as a snack or for adding to a basic salad to spice it up.

Place the mango and avocado in a bowl with the red onion, chilli, olive oil, lime juice and coriander and mix to combine. Season to taste with salt and pepper, then cover the bowl with a plate and leave to stand at room temperature for 15 minutes to let the flavours blend before serving.

Stored in the fridge in an airtight container, the salsa can be kept for up to 1 day before the avocado begins to go brown.

Serves 4

360g cherry tomatoes
(or 6 large tomatoes),
finely chopped
½ red onion, finely diced
1 tbsp fresh lime juice

Salt and black pepper
Handful of coriander,
chopped, to garnish

Cherry Tomato Salsa

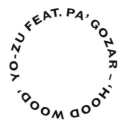

A fresh and flavourful cherry tomato salsa made with garlic, lime, red onions and coriander. This classic salsa is a great party dip, and perfect in wraps, fajitas, burritos and tacos.

In a bowl, mix the tomatoes with the red onion. Add the lime juice and season to taste with salt and pepper, then garnish with a sprinkling of the coriander to serve.

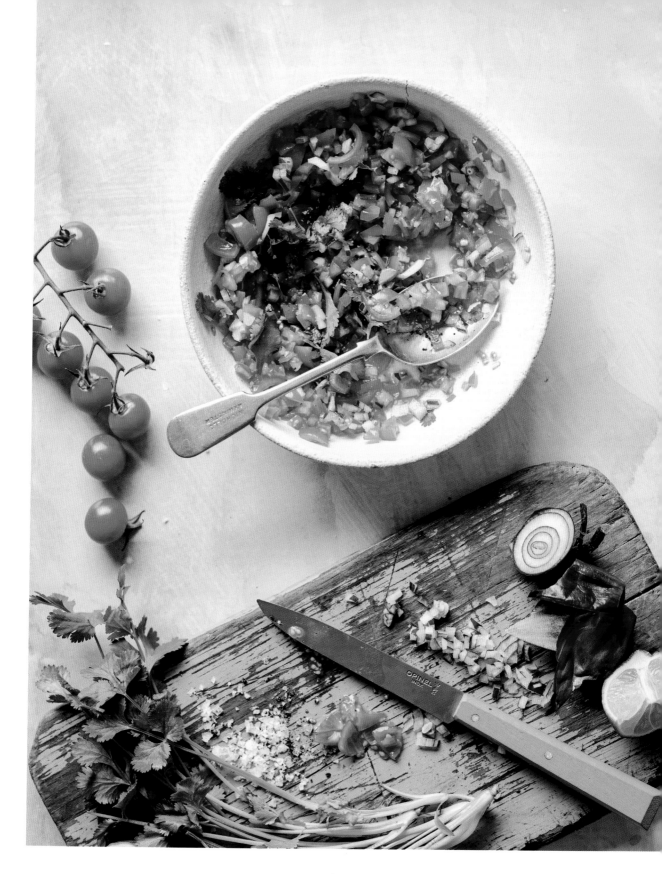

2 tbsp olive oil

2 red onions, sliced

½ quantity Roast Red
    Peppers (see page 154)
    or 2 roasted red peppers
    in oil (from a jar), drained
    and roughly chopped

100g sun-dried tomatoes,
    roughly chopped

1 tsp ground sumac

Juice and grated zest of
    ½ lemon

1 tbsp pomegranate
    molasses

Small handful of
    fresh parsley leaves,
    finely chopped

Salt and black pepper

Red Onion and Red Pepper Salsa

Sweet roast red peppers and caramelised red onions mixed together with umami sun-dried tomatoes and a touch of sumac make for a really flavourful salsa. It's good in a sandwich and as a dipping side for roast vegetables or baby potatoes.

Place 1 tablespoon of the oil in a small non-stick frying pan, then add the onions and cook over a medium heat for 7–10 minutes, stirring occasionally, until soft, caramelised and sticky. Remove from the heat and allow to cool slightly before tipping them on to a board and roughly chopping them.

Add the chopped onions to a bowl with the remaining ingredients. Mix together well and season to taste with salt and pepper. Serve immediately or store in the fridge in an airtight container for up to a week.

Sides, Sauces and Dips

Makes 200ml

6 spring onions,
    roughly chopped
Thumb-sized piece of fresh
    root ginger, peeled and
    roughly chopped
½–2 fresh red Scotch
    bonnet chillies (to taste),
    deseeded and roughly
    chopped
4 garlic cloves,
    roughly chopped

1 tbsp fresh thyme leaves
60ml extra-virgin olive oil
3 tbsp soy sauce
    (or coconut aminos)
Juice of 1 lime
½ tsp ground nutmeg
1 tbsp ground allspice
1 tbsp vegan
    white wine vinegar
1 tbsp coconut sugar
Salt and black pepper

Jerk Marinade

When people think of jerk, they often think jerk chicken, but the jerk is all about the seasoning. I love using this marinade for brushing on griddled vegetables like cauliflower and especially for making the Jerk Mushroom and Caramelised Onion Feast on page 138. If you are not used to cooking and eating Scotch bonnet, start off with a small amount as it is spicy!

Place all the ingredients in a food processor and blitz into a rough paste, seasoning to taste with salt and pepper. The marinade can be stored in the fridge in an airtight container for up to 4 days.

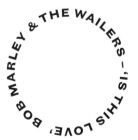

BOB MARLEY & THE WAILERS – 'IS THIS LOVE'

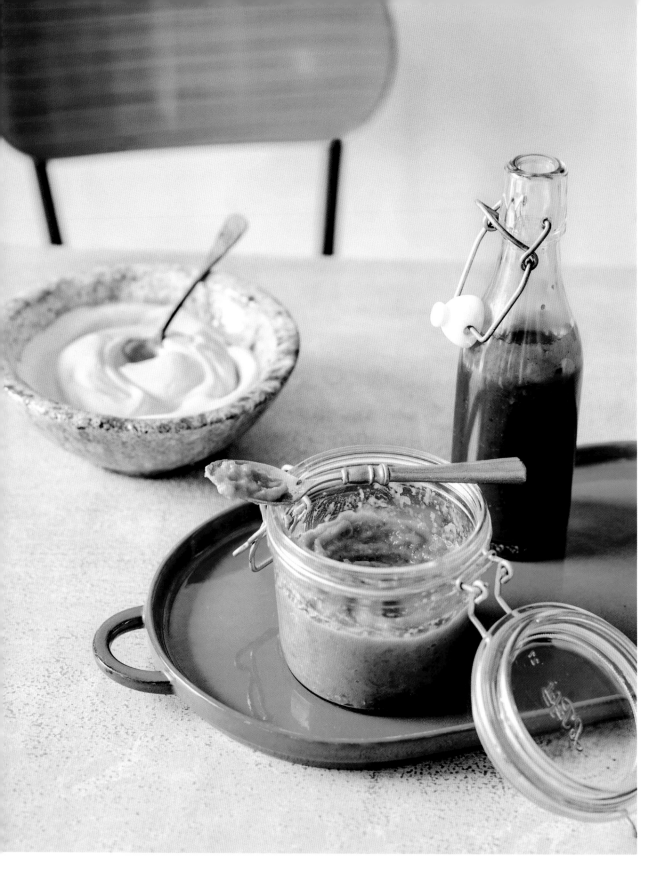

Sides, Sauces and Dips

Makes about 900ml

Thumb-sized piece
    of fresh root ginger,
    peeled and grated
3 garlic cloves,
    finely chopped
4 spring onions,
    roughly chopped
½ fresh red Scotch bonnet
    chilli, deseeded and
    roughly chopped

Leaves from 3 thyme sprigs
1 tbsp vegetable oil
1 tsp ground nutmeg
1 tsp ground cinnamon
1 tbsp ground allspice
480ml tomato ketchup
100ml water
60ml soy sauce
    (or coconut aminos)

1 tbsp vegan
    white wine vinegar
1 tbsp vegan
    Worcestershire sauce
3–5 tbsp maple syrup
1 tbsp liquid smoke (or soy
    sauce or coconut aminos)
1 tsp English mustard
Salt and black pepper

Jerk Barbecue Sauce

The fiery Caribbean spices of traditional jerk seasoning are combined here with a touch of sweetness and little kick from the Scotch bonnet chilli to create this delicious barbecue sauce (it's on the far right in the photo opposite). It's perfect for brushing on griddled vegetables in the summertime, or for serving with vegan meat substitutes. I absolutely love this with my Jerk Aubergine Burgers and Crispy Jerk Barbecue Tacos (see pages 131 and 127)!

Place the ginger and garlic in blender or food processor with the spring onions, chilli and thyme and blitz into a rough paste.

Place the vegetable oil in a deep frying pan and add the paste and all the spices. Season with salt and pepper and sauté over a low heat for about 5 minutes until the paste starts to brown.

Add all the remaining ingredients, using the smaller quantity of maple syrup. Mix to combine and then cook for 15 minutes on a low heat, stirring occasionally, until the sauce thickens. Taste, and add more of the maple syrup if needed. Remove from the heat and allow to cool before serving.

If not using immediately, the sauce can be stored in the fridge in an airtight container for up to 4 days, which allows it time to mature and develop its best flavour.

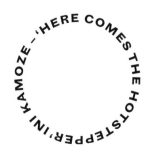

INI KAMOZE – 'HERE COMES THE HOTSTEPPER'

Makes about 550ml

1 tbsp vegetable oil
1 red onion, finely diced
3 garlic cloves, finely
    chopped
¼ fresh red Scotch bonnet
    chilli, deseeded and
    roughly chopped
    (optional, for heat)
1 tbsp grated
    fresh root ginger

1 tbsp tomato purée
160g mango flesh,
    roughly chopped
160g pineapple flesh,
    roughly chopped
2 tbsp maple syrup
    (optional, for sweetness)
2 tbsp fresh lime juice
1 tsp apple cider vinegar
Salt and black pepper

Mango Pineapple Ketchup

Made with fresh mango and pineapple for a fun twist on standard tomato ketchup, this is a great accompaniment to burgers, such as the Jerk Aubergine Burgers on page 131. Use as a substitute for regular ketchup when you want a tropical twist! See photo (centre) on page 186.

Pour the vegetable oil into a small saucepan, add the onion and garlic and fry over a medium heat for 5–10 minutes until soft and lightly caramelised. Transfer to a plate and leave to cool.

Once the onion mixture has cooled down, place in a food processor with all the remaining ingredients and blend to a smooth purée, seasoning to taste with salt and pepper.

Pour the purée into a heavy-based saucepan and simmer over a low heat for up to 1 hour until thickened. Allow to cool, then transfer to a bowl and chill in the fridge for at least an hour before using. The ketchup can be kept in an airtight container in the fridge for up to 3 days.

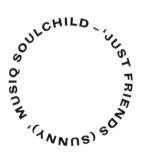

MUSIQ SOULCHILD – 'JUST FRIENDS (SUNNY)'

Makes about 610ml

120ml aquafaba (liquid
    from a tin of chickpeas)
½ tsp English
    mustard powder
½ tsp garlic granules
1 tsp fresh lemon juice

480ml rapeseed oil
    (or extra-virgin olive
    oil or avocado oil)
Salt (or black salt)
    and black pepper

Aquafaba Mayo

A vegan, completely soy-free alternative to mayonnaise that still tastes like the genuine article! It is also one of my favourite ways of using aquafaba (the cooking liquid from chickpeas and other legumes, see page 242). My favourite type of aquafaba is the water from a tin of chickpeas, which I've suggested using here. The sulphur compounds in Himalayan black salt create an egg-like flavour that's reminiscent of classic mayonnaise, but whether you use this or standard table salt is entirely up to you. See photo on page 186 (left).

Place the aquafaba, mustard, garlic and lemon juice in a high-speed blender, season with salt and pepper and blend until frothy. Alternatively, mix all the ingredients using a hand blender.

While blending at high speed, slowly pour in the oil bit by bit over a period of 3–5 minutes and blend until thick and creamy. Taste for seasoning, adding more salt and pepper if needed.

Transfer the mayo to a bowl, then cover with a plate and chill in the fridge for an hour until cold and to allow it to get even thicker before serving. The mayo can be stored in the fridge in an airtight container for up to 3 days.

125ml soya milk,
    at room temperature
1 tsp vegan
    white wine vinegar
1 tsp fresh lemon juice
½ tsp yellow mustard powder
¼ tsp garlic granules
250ml extra-virgin avocado
    oil (or rapeseed oil)
Salt (or black salt)
    and black pepper

Soy Mayo

An incredibly quick recipe for whipping up a delicious vegan mayo in 5 minutes – it looks and tastes just like your regular mayonnaise! You can make it even thicker by adding more oil bit by bit but I find this consistency perfect. It is important for the milk and oil to be at room temperature before combining so that they emulsify into a mayonnaise. You will need either a high-speed blender or a stick blender to make this mayo.

Place the milk in a high-speed blender with the vinegar, lemon juice and mustard powder, season with salt and pepper and then blend until smooth. Alternatively, mix all the ingredients using a hand blender.

While blending at high speed, gradually pour in the oil over a period of 2–3 minutes until thick and creamy. Taste for seasoning, adding more salt and pepper if needed.

Pour the mayo into a sterilised jar (see page 175), seal with a lid and chill in the fridge before serving. The mayo can be kept in the jar in the fridge for up to 3 days.

Serves 4

2 tbsp gherkins,
    drained and finely
    chopped
1 garlic clove, finely chopped
2 tbsp drained capers,
    finely chopped
1 tbsp finely chopped parsley

1 tsp English mustard
220ml vegan mayonnaise
    (to make your own,
    see page 189 or 190)
1 tbsp fresh lemon juice
Salt and black pepper

Tartare Sauce

A must-have with Beer-battered Aubergine and Chips (see page 119)! Sharp and tangy with gherkins, capers and freshly squeezed lemon.

Place all the ingredients in a bowl and mix well to combine, seasoning to taste with salt and pepper. If not using immediately, this can be stored in the fridge in an airtight container for up to a week.

Thumb-sized piece of
fresh root ginger, peeled
and finely chopped
1 garlic clove, finely chopped
200g smooth natural peanut
butter (to make your own,
see page 240)

2 tbsp soy sauce
(or coconut aminos)
1 tbsp fresh lime juice
2 tbsp maple syrup
1 tbsp harissa paste
120ml warm water
1 tbsp vegan
rice wine vinegar

Peanut Sauce

Made with fresh ginger and lime juice, a hint of spice and a touch of maple syrup for sweetness, this is a super-simple sauce yet so versatile too. I love to use it for making Peanut Fried Rice (see page 168), for adding to noodle dishes or even for drizzling over crunchy veg, such as cabbage, carrots and peppers!

Place all the ingredients in a bowl and whisk into a smooth sauce. Transfer to a clean, lidded jar and store in the fridge for up to 2 days for the best flavour. The sauce can thicken slightly over time, so add a splash of water to loosen, if needed.

Makes 300ml

2 nori sheets
240ml water
60ml soy sauce
  (or coconut aminos)
1 tbsp shiitake powder
1 tbsp brown miso paste
1 tsp garlic granules
1 tsp vegan rice wine vinegar

Vegan Fish Sauce

Perfect for recipes that traditionally call for fish sauce. I love throwing this into stir-fries – the miso paste adds an extra depth of flavour combined with sea-like essence from the nori sheets. I like to make a quick batch on a Monday and then add it to my recipes throughout the week.

Place all the ingredients in a food processor and blend until the nori sheets have combined with the liquid to make a smooth sauce. Keep stored in the fridge in an airtight container for up to a week.

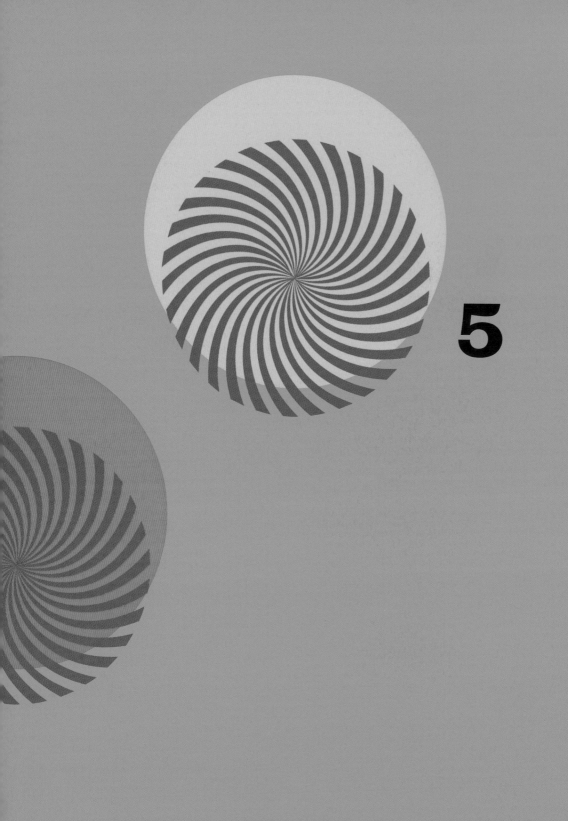

5

PUDDINGS

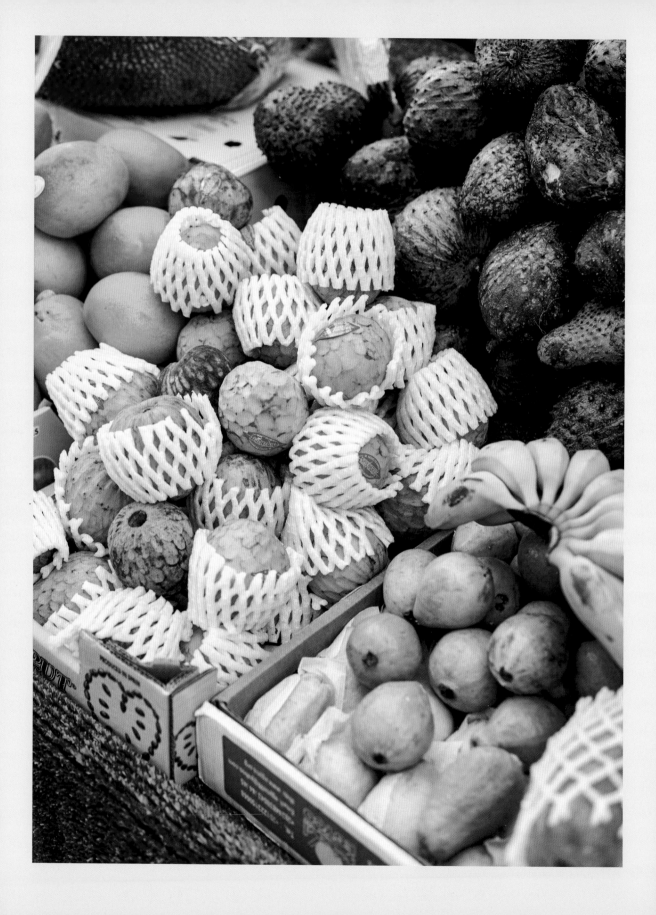

Puddings

When it comes to puddings and desserts my heart is always set on chocolate and cakes so in this chapter you'll find chocolate fudge brownies, crumbles and ginger cake. The lemon drizzle cake is a particular favourite, especially with a cup of tea. But with summer in mind, there are also recipes for grilled fruits with sticky nut toppings and ice cream, as well as simple tropical chia seed lollies.

I love meringue so I couldn't not have a pavlova recipe, made with fresh berries (or seasonal fruit of your choice) and whipped coconut cream – it's a real showstopper if you are hosting any summer parties.

Vegan baking is a little different to regular baking, but fear not, there are a few different ways to replace the eggs in traditional baking (see my suggestions on page 236 and 237) to keep your cakes light, soft and moist!

When it comes to replacing butter my favourite option is rapeseed oil – it is rich and buttery and works amazingly well in cakes and other bakes.

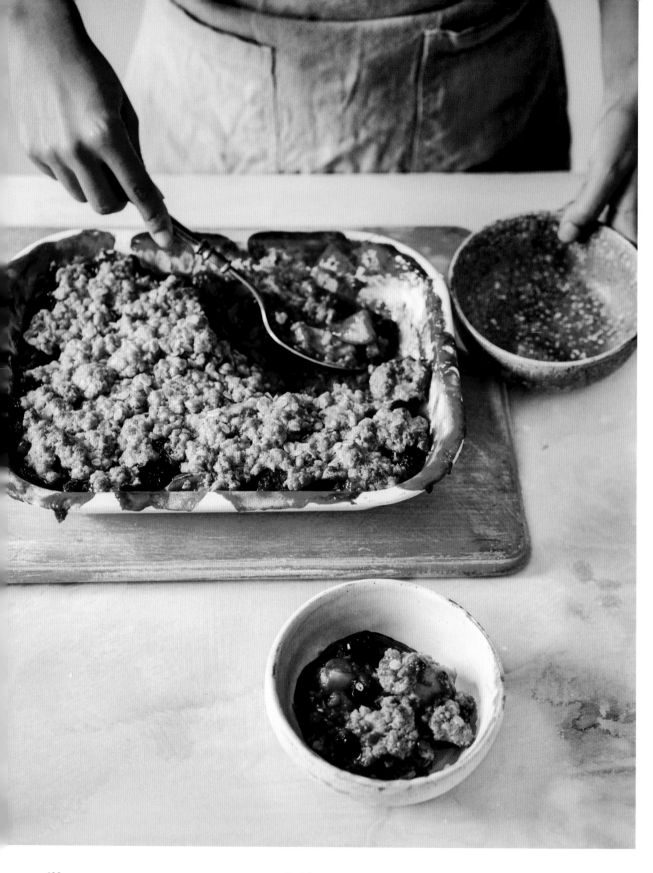

Puddings

Serves 8

500g Granny Smith apples (about 6 apples), peeled, cored and diced into small cubes
250g fresh or frozen (and defrosted) raspberries
250g fresh or frozen (and defrosted) blueberries
45g soft light brown sugar
1 tsp ground cinnamon
1 tbsp fresh lemon juice
60ml water
3 tbsp plain flour

For the crumble

130g plain flour
1 tsp ground cinnamon
Pinch of salt
50g ground almonds
90g rolled oats
100g coconut sugar
210g chilled vegan butter or coconut oil

To serve

Vegan vanilla ice cream or custard

You will need a 2–3-litre baking dish

Apple Berry Crumble

My favourite dessert when I was growing up was apple crumble with custard and this is my vegan take on it. Get stuck into the crunchy and sweet crumble with tender apples and juicy berries. I feel there's a real divide between those who like crumble with custard and those who prefer it with ice cream. I've recently discovered a third group: people who like it with both custard *and* ice cream – mind blown! But however you like your crumble, it's still one of the most comforting desserts.

'MAZE (FEAT. FRANKIE BEVERLY) – 'WE ARE ONE'

Preheat the oven to 180°C fan.

Place the apples, raspberries and blueberries in a deep, heavy-based saucepan. Add the sugar, cinnamon, lemon juice and water and mix together gently to combine. Add the flour and then cook over a low heat for 5 minutes to soften slightly, stirring occasionally and taking care not to break up the fruit.

For the crumble, sift the flour, cinnamon and salt into a large bowl, then add the ground almonds, oats and sugar and mix to combine.

Add the butter and rub in with your fingertips until light and breadcrumb-like in texture. Try not to overwork the mixture or the cooked crumble will be heavy.

Spoon the cooked apples and berries into the baking dish, then cover with the crumble mixture. Bake in the oven for about 40 minutes until the filling is bubbling and the topping is golden brown. Keep an eye on it during cooking to make sure it doesn't burn.

Remove from the oven and serve with vegan vanilla ice cream or custard.

1 ripe pineapple
2 tbsp maple syrup
1 tbsp ground cinnamon
1 tbsp vegetable oil

For the salted caramel sauce
240ml maple syrup
2 tbsp vegan butter
60ml vegan cream
1–2 pinches of salt (to taste)

To serve
4 scoops of vegan coconut ice cream
125g pecans, lightly crushed

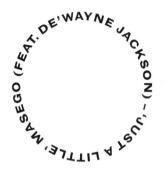

MASEGO (FEAT. DE'WAYNE JACKSON) – 'JUST A LITTLE'

Griddled Cinnamon Pineapples with Salted Caramel

Here, juicy pineapples are marinated in maple and cinnamon and then griddled until caramelised before being drizzled with salted caramel sauce and crunchy pecans and served with coconut ice cream. The pineapples are also amazing cooked on the barbecue in the summer.

First make the salted caramel sauce. Pour the maple syrup into a non-stick saucepan set over a medium heat and bring to a gentle boil, then allow the syrup to bubble away for about 15 minutes. Stir occasionally with a wooden spoon to reduce the bubbles.

Add the butter and stir until it has completely melted. Whisking the sauce constantly, gradually add the cream until it has all been combined. Add the salt and mix in well, then pour the sauce into a jar or bowl and set aside to cool.

Meanwhile, place the pineapple on a chopping board on its side and, using a large sharp knife, slice off the base of the fruit and the green top – cutting through the pineapple 1–2cm from the base of the leaves. Stand the pineapple up and begin to carefully slice away the outer peel, cutting from top to bottom and following the contours of the pineapple. Lay the pineapple on its side and cut into 5cm slices.

Place the pineapple in a large bowl, then add the maple syrup and cinnamon and stir to coat the pineapple evenly. Leave to marinate for about 30 minutes.

Place a griddle pan (or a heavy-based frying pan) over a medium heat and add the vegetable oil. Add the pineapple slices and cook for about 5 minutes on each side or until heated through and lightly chargrilled. Divide the griddled pineapples between plates and serve with a generous scoop of coconut ice cream, a drizzle of the salted caramel sauce and a sprinkling of crushed pecans.

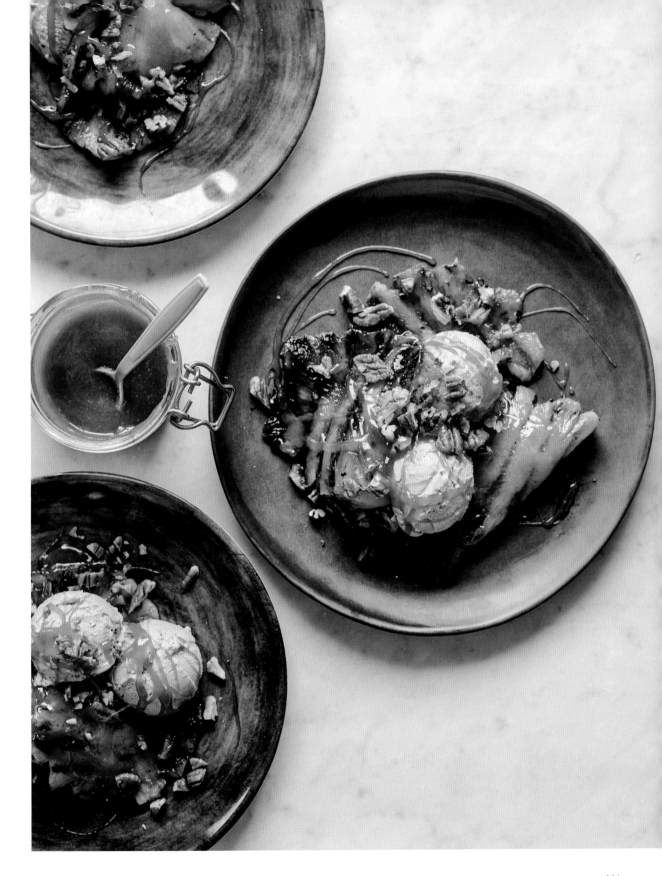

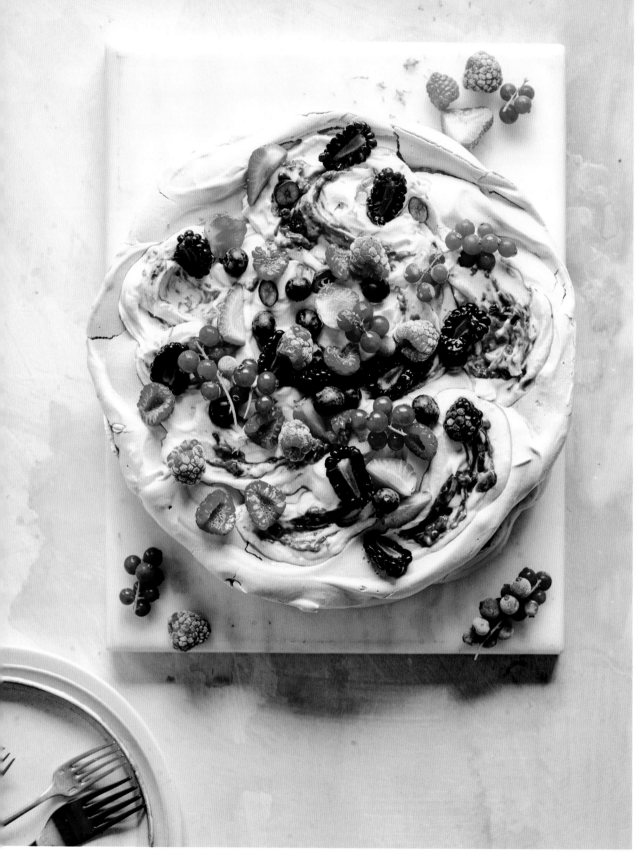

Puddings

Serves 6

For the meringue

Liquid (aquafaba) from
  1 × 400g tin of chickpeas
1 tsp cream of tartar
175g golden caster sugar
1 tsp vanilla bean paste

For the filling and topping

500ml coconut cream
200g mixed frozen berries
Juice and grated zest of
  ½ lime, plus extra zest
  to decorate
300g seasonal fruit of
  your choice (such as
  raspberries, strawberries,
  blueberries or
  redcurrants, sliced figs,
  mangos or bananas or
  passion fruit pulp)

Layered Pavlova with Coconut Cream

Your summer-party showstopping recipe! The meringue is made with aquafaba instead of egg whites. You may or may not be familiar with aquafaba: it is the liquid from a can of pulses. It's kind of like vegan magic; it whips up perfectly and makes amazing light meringues with a slight crisp outer shell (for more about it see page 242). The pavlova is finished with an indulgent whipped coconut cream, fresh or frozen berries and a tasty and decorative berry drizzle.

Preheat the oven to 130°C fan, then line two baking sheets with baking paper and draw a 23cm circle on each sheet.

Place the coconut cream in the fridge to chill while you make the meringue.

Using a food mixer or an electric whisk, whisk the aquafaba and cream of tartar at a high speed in a large bowl for around 5 minutes until the mixture has doubled in volume and is light and fluffy.

Continue whisking and add the sugar 1 teaspoon at a time until it has been completely absorbed. Then add the vanilla bean paste and whisk for a further 2 minutes until the mixture forms stiff, glossy peaks.

Divide the meringue between the two circles drawn on the lined baking sheets, spreading the mixture out evenly but making each circle a little thicker around the edges than in the middle. Place in the oven to cook for 1½–1¾ hours or until firm to the touch, then turn off the heat and leave to dry in the oven (or in a cool, dry place) overnight or for a minimum of 4 hours.

Continued on the next page

ANGIE STONE (FEAT. MUSIQ SOULCHILD) – 'THE INGREDIENTS OF LOVE'

When the meringues are ready, prepare the rest of the dish. Place the frozen berries and lime juice in a small saucepan, bring to a simmer and cook on a medium heat for 3–4 minutes or until the fruit is soft and the liquid has mostly evaporated. Remove from the heat and set aside to cool down completely.

Meanwhile, whisk the chilled coconut cream using an electric whisk until light and thick like whipped cream. Once the fruit compote has cooled down, add it to the whipped coconut cream with the lime zest, and fold in gently to create a ripple effect, being careful not to stir too much.

Carefully transfer one of the meringue bases to a serving plate and spread over half the fruity coconut cream, then scatter over half the seasonal fruit. Carefully place the second meringue on top, cover with the remaining coconut cream and seasonal fruit and an extra sprinkling of lime zest. Serve as soon as possible.

Serves 4

2 nectarines, cut into
     wedges 3cm thick
2 tbsp maple syrup
Juice and finely grated
     zest of 1 lime

For the praline
250g caster sugar
175g mixed nuts (such as
     almonds, pecans and
     pistachios)

To serve
Vegan coconut ice cream

Maple Pan-fried Nectarines with Nut Praline

The sweet and crunchy praline is so incredibly addictive and goes brilliantly with warm and sticky nectarines fried in maple syrup and lime juice. Of course, a side of coconut ice cream brings it all together.

To make the praline, first line a baking sheet with baking paper. Place the sugar in a heavy-based saucepan set over a low heat and allow it to melt slowly for about 5 minutes, shaking the pan occasionally to ensure that it melts evenly. Keep an eye on the sugar as it caramelises until it's glossy and golden. Don't be tempted to stir the mixture or dip your finger in to test it – it will be extremely hot!

When all the sugar has melted and is glossy and golden, add the nuts and quickly stir until they are fully coated and then immediately pour the mixture onto the prepared baking sheet. Allow to cool completely before breaking into small pieces. Or, you can blitz the praline in a food processor to a finer crumb, if you prefer.

Place the nectarine wedges in a dry non-stick frying pan and cook over a high heat for 1 minute on each side until starting to brown. Reduce the heat, add the maple syrup and lime juice and cook for another 1–2 minutes on each side until softened, sticky and caramelised.

Divide between bowls and serve scattered with the lime zest and praline and with a scoop of coconut ice cream.

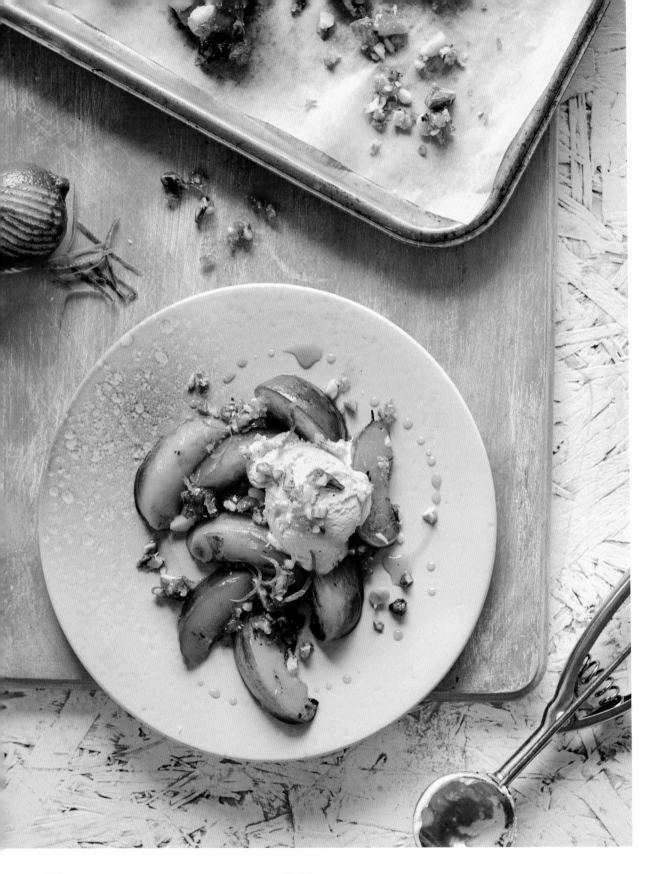

Puddings

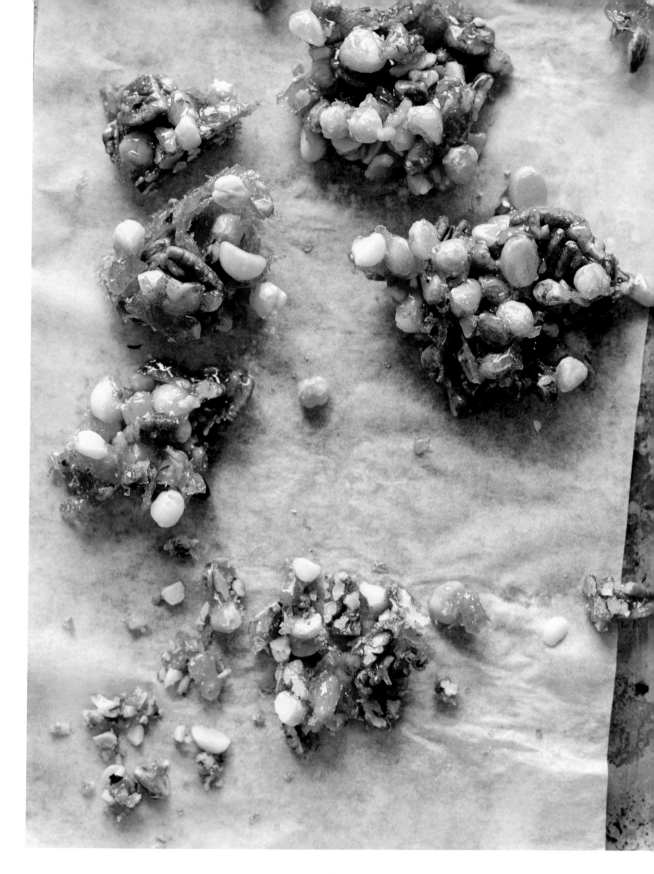

Makes 8–10 ice lollies

1 ripe mango,
 roughly chopped
120ml coconut water
3–4 tbsp maple syrup
1 tsp chia seeds
240g unsweetened vegan
 coconut yoghurt
Pulp and seeds of
 2 passion fruit

**You will need an
8–10-hole ice-lolly
mould and 8–10 sticks**

Mango Chia Seed Passion Fruit Ice Lollies

Sweet and refreshing mango purée is mixed with nutritious chia seeds and creamy coconut yoghurt and popped in the freezer to create these amazing tropical lollies! Perfect on a summer's day for cooling you down.

Place the mango and coconut water in a blender or food processor and purée until smooth. Transfer to a bowl and taste. If the mango isn't quite ripe and sweet enough, then add 1–2 tablespoons of the maple syrup to taste, and fold in the chia seeds.

Mix together the yoghurt and remaining maple syrup, then fold in the passion fruit pulp and seeds.

Pour in enough of the mango purée to fill each lolly mould by one-third, then fill to the top with the passion fruit and yoghurt mixture. Place in the freezer to set for 1 hour, then insert a lolly stick into each mould and return to the freezer to set completely. To remove the lollies, dip the moulds in hot water before carefully removing each lolly from its mould.

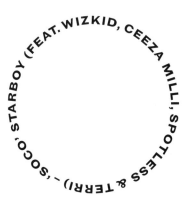
'SOCO', STARBOY (FEAT. WIZKID, CEEZA MILLI, SPOTLESS & TERRI)

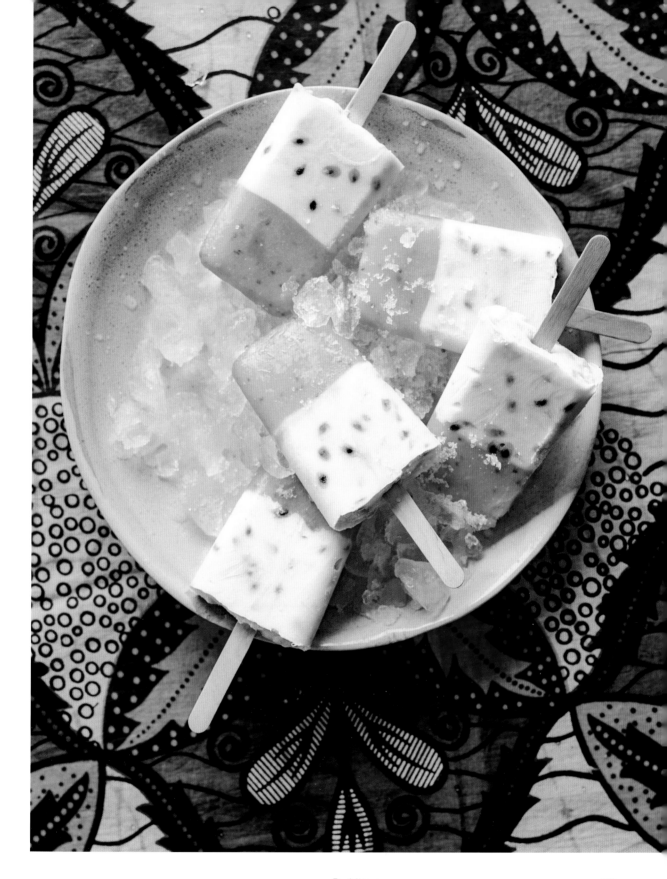

Makes 1 loaf

8 dates, pitted
3 ripe bananas, peeled
90g coconut oil, melted,
    plus extra for greasing
1 tbsp vanilla extract
1 tbsp apple cider vinegar
90g plain flour
1 tsp baking powder
1 tsp bicarbonate of soda
½ tsp ground cinnamon
Pinch of salt
90g wholemeal flour
2 flax eggs (see page 236)

To serve (optional)
Vegan butter
Chia Raspberry Jam
    (see page 35)

**You will need one
900g loaf tin**

Banana Bread

Simple, soft and moist, this banana loaf is completely addictive. I love a warm slice of banana bread as a snack at any time of day. Sometimes I spread it with vegan butter and chia jam, just like a piece of toast, or with nut butter (see page 240). For the best results, make sure you use ripe bananas that are sweet and soft.

Preheat the oven to 175°C fan, then grease the loaf tin with coconut oil and line with baking paper.

Place the dates in a bowl of warm water for 10 minutes to soften them. Drain and add to a food processor with the bananas, then blend into a coarse paste.

Pour the date and banana paste into a bowl and mix in the melted coconut oil, vanilla extract and apple cider vinegar. In a separate bowl, sift together the plain flour, baking powder, bicarbonate of soda, cinnamon and salt, then add the wholemeal flour.

Add the wet ingredients to the bowl with the dry ingredients, then fold in the flax eggs, and mix together well to combine.

Pour the batter into the prepared loaf tin and bake in the oven for 50 minutes or until a skewer inserted into the centre of the loaf comes out clean. Remove from the oven and allow to cool for a few minutes before removing from the tin and transferring to a wire rack to cool down completely.

Cut into slices and spread with vegan butter and/or chia raspberry jam, if you like. The banana bread can be stored for up to 3 days in a tin or other airtight container.

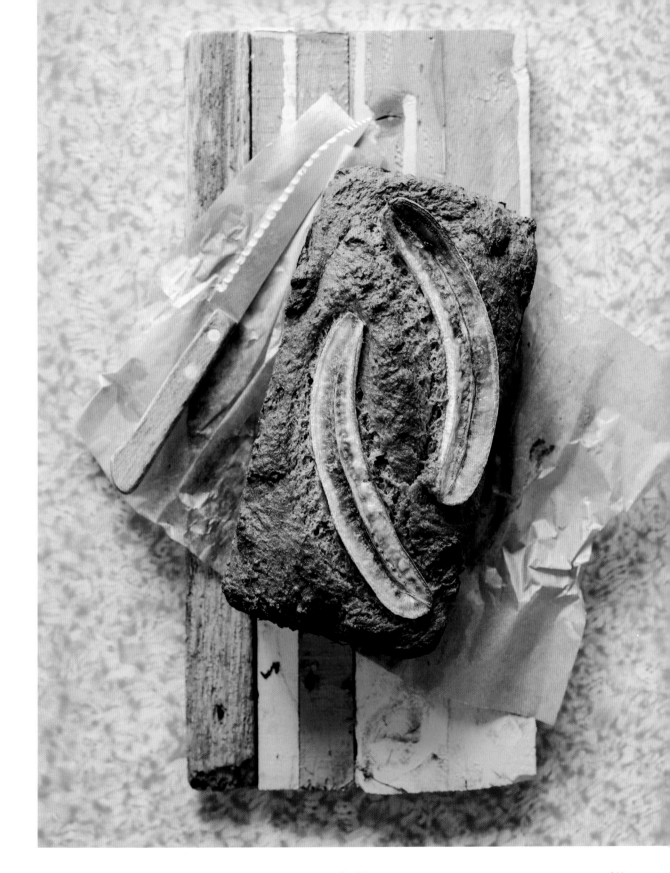

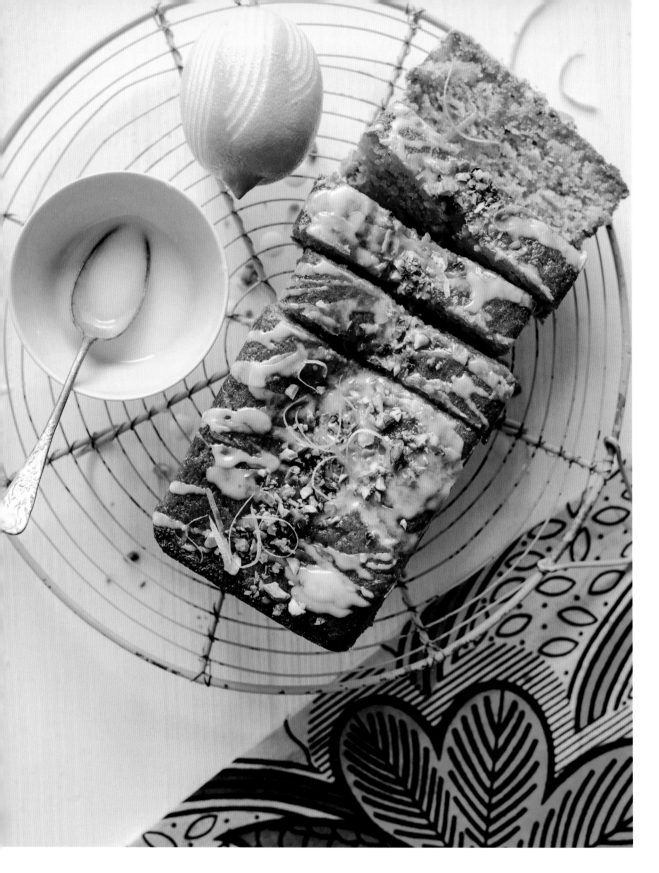

Puddings

Serves 8–10

245ml plant-based milk
(to make your own,
see page 238)
5 tbsp fresh lemon juice
200g golden caster sugar
75ml extra-virgin rapeseed
oil (or coconut oil),
plus extra for greasing
2 tsp vanilla extract
Grated zest of 1 lemon

160g plain flour
¼ tsp bicarbonate of soda
1 tsp baking powder
Pinch of salt
90g ground almonds

For the lemon syrup
Juice of 2 lemons
1 tbsp maple syrup

For the topping
75g icing sugar, sifted
1–2 tbsp fresh lemon juice
Handful of pistachios,
roughly crushed

You will need
a 900g loaf tin

Lemon and Almond Drizzle Cake with Pistachios

Made with ground almonds that keep it extra moist, and topped with a tangy lemon icing and pistachio nuts, this cake is a real classic. What better way to enjoy the afternoon than with a cup of tea and a slice of this decadent lemon drizzle cake? Use unwaxed lemons if you can.

Preheat the oven to 180°C fan, then grease the loaf tin with rapeseed oil and line with baking paper.

Combine the milk with 1 tablespoon of the lemon juice and set aside for 10 minutes to curdle.

In a large bowl, whisk together the sugar and rapeseed oil to combine. Use an electric whisk for this, if you can. Pour in the curdled milk with the vanilla extract, lemon zest and remaining 4 tablespoons of lemon juice, and whisk together.

Sift the plain flour into a separate bowl with the bicarbonate of soda, baking powder and salt and then add the ground almonds. Add the dry ingredients to the batter and fold in gently to combine.

Transfer the batter to the prepared loaf tin and bake in the oven for about 40 minutes until a skewer inserted into the middle of the cake comes out clean.

Meanwhile, combine the lemon juice and maple syrup.

When the cake is baked, remove from the oven and the baking tin, place on a wire rack and then pierce the top in several places with a skewer, cover in the lemon syrup and leave the cake to cool down completely.

Whisk together the icing sugar and lemon juice until smooth, then drizzle over the cooled cake and decorate with the crushed pistachios. Store for up to 3 days in a tin or other airtight container.

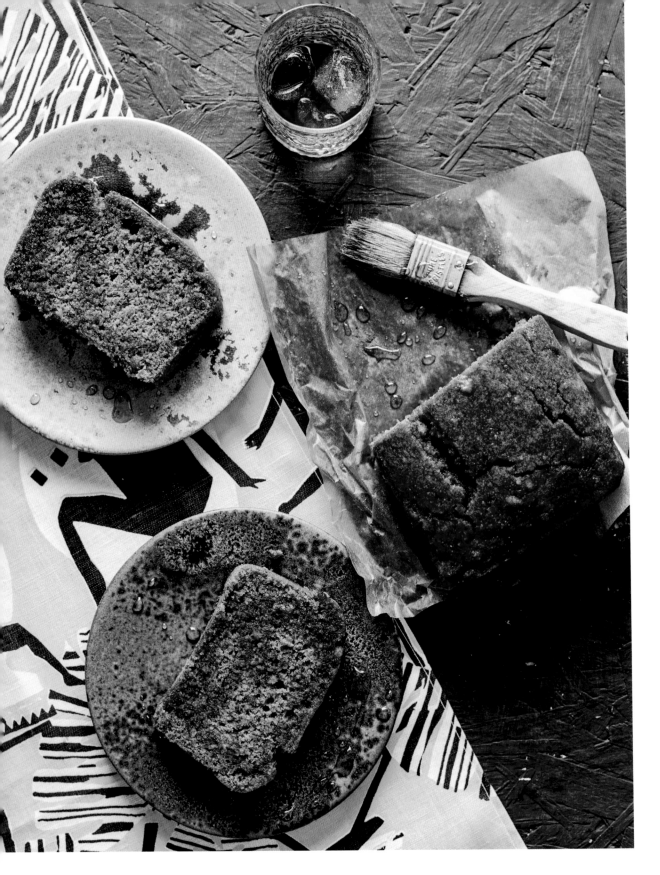

Puddings

Serves 8–10

2 tbsp dark muscovado sugar

80ml maple syrup, plus
  2–3 tbsp for drizzling

170g full-fat coconut milk

60g fresh root ginger, peeled
  and very finely chopped
  into a purée (or 80g stem
  ginger, finely chopped)

75ml extra-virgin rapeseed
  oil (or coconut oil or
  vegan butter), plus extra
  for greasing

1 tsp vanilla extract

110g plain flour

1 tsp bicarbonate of soda

1 tsp baking powder

1 tsp ground cinnamon

½ tsp ground allspice

1 tbsp ground ginger

Pinch of salt

110g wholemeal flour

2 flax eggs (see page 236)

1 tbsp fresh lemon juice

**You will need
a 900g loaf tin**

Spiced
Ginger Cake

Popular in the Caribbean, this spiced ginger cake is warming and tasty. And with a sticky maple glaze on top, it's hard to stop going back for more! I like to use fresh root ginger because it's easier to get hold of – I always have some in the house and it hasn't got added sugars, but you can substitute it with stem ginger if you prefer.

Preheat the oven to 180°C fan, then grease the loaf tin with rapeseed oil and line with baking paper.

In a large bowl, whisk together the sugar, maple syrup, coconut milk, ginger, rapeseed oil and vanilla extract.

In a separate bowl, sift together the plain flour, bicarbonate of soda, baking powder, spices and salt, then add the wholemeal flour.

Gently fold the wet ingredients into the flour mixture and mix to combine. Fold in the flax eggs, then add the lemon juice and gently mix in.

Transfer the batter to the prepared loaf tin and bake in the oven for 40 minutes or until a skewer inserted into the middle of the cake comes out clean.

Remove from the oven, leave to cool in the tin for 5 minutes, then remove from the tin and transfer to a wire rack to cool completely. Once cooled, drizzle over the maple syrup and cut into slices to serve. This cake can be stored in a tin or other airtight container for up to 4 days.

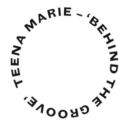

TEENA MARIE – 'BEHIND THE GROOVE'

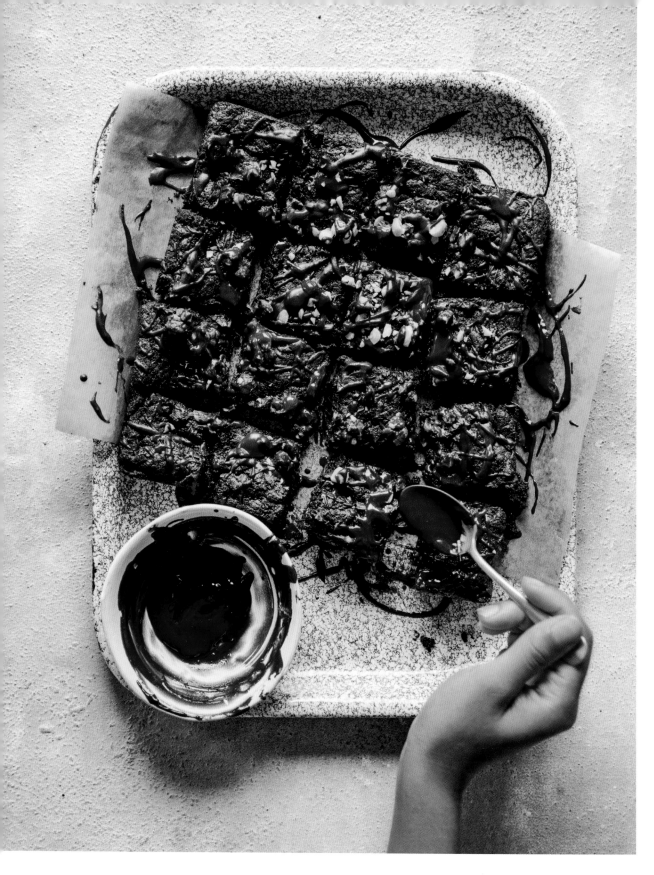

Puddings

Makes 16 brownies

170g vegan dark chocolate

200g soft dark brown sugar

80g extra-virgin rapeseed oil,
    plus extra for greasing

2 tsp vanilla extract

95g plain flour

30g cocoa powder

1 tsp baking powder

Pinch of salt

2 flax eggs (see page 236)

For the hazelnut swirl

Handful of whole hazelnuts

50g vegan dark chocolate,
    broken into squares

1 tbsp maple syrup

1 tbsp coconut oil, melted

Pinch of salt

**You will need a 23cm
square cake tin**

Fudgy Chocolate Brownies with Hazelnut Swirl

For a self-confessed chocolate lover, these rich and fudgy brownies are so very satisfying! They're best eaten while they're still slightly warm from the oven so you get to enjoy the gooeyness with the melted chocolate chunks for the perfect chocolate overload. The brownies are quite soft in the middle when they come out of the oven (the melted chocolate doing its thang). If you prefer a more solid brownie, just leave them to cool down fully. And don't forget that generous pinch of salt to intensify the chocolate flavour!

Preheat the oven to 180°C fan, then grease the tin with rapeseed oil and line the base with baking paper.

Take 110g of the chocolate and break it into squares. Fill a saucepan with water to a depth of 2–3cm and bring to a simmer, then reduce the heat to low. Place the chocolate in a heatproof bowl that will fit snugly on top of the pan without the simmering water touching the base of the bowl. Stir the chocolate occasionally as it begins to soften, then remove the pan from the heat once the chocolate has melted. Chop the rest of the chocolate into rough chunks.

Place the brown sugar and rapeseed oil in a large bowl and whisk until smooth. Add the vanilla extract and the melted chocolate and whisk again until smooth.

Sift the flour, cocoa powder, baking powder and salt into a separate bowl, then combine with the oil and chocolate mixture. Fold in the flax eggs – taking care not to over-mix – and then fold in the chocolate chunks.

Pour the batter into the prepared cake tin and smooth the surface with a spatula. Bake for 30 minutes, until a skewer inserted in the middle comes out with just a little oil on it.

Continued on the next page

Remove from the oven and allow to cool in the tin for
5 minutes, then transfer from the tin to a wire rack and
leave to cool for 20 minutes.

Meanwhile, spread the hazelnuts on a baking tray and
roast in the oven for 5–10 minutes, tossing them halfway
through and checking regularly to ensure that they don't
burn. Remove from the oven, place on a clean tea towel
and gently rub to remove the skins. Allow to cool, then
roughly crush with a rolling pin or the base of a heavy pan.

Melt the 50g of chocolate as before in a heatproof
bowl over a pan of just-simmering water, then mix with
the crushed hazelnuts, maple syrup, melted coconut
oil and salt. Stir well to combine and then pour on
top of the cooled brownies.

Slice into squares and serve. These are best eaten
while still slightly warm. If not eating immediately,
store in a tin or other airtight container for up to 3 days.
The brownies can be reheated in the oven to get warm
and fudgy again.

MJ COLE AND KOJEY RADICAL – 'SOAK IT UP'

Makes 10–12 cupcakes

120g plain flour
1 tsp baking powder
1 tsp bicarbonate of soda
2 tsp ground cinnamon
½ tsp ground nutmeg
Pinch of salt
120g wholemeal flour
200g carrots, peeled
   and grated
200g soft dark brown sugar
120ml extra-virgin
   rapeseed oil

120ml plant-based milk
   (to make your own,
   see page 238)
1 tsp vanilla extract
2 flax eggs (see page 236)
1 tbsp fresh lemon juice
Handful of walnut pieces,
   crushed, to decorate

For the frosting
450g icing sugar, sifted
3 tbsp coconut oil, melted
1 tsp vanilla extract
2 tsp apple cider vinegar
3–4 tbsp fresh lemon juice
1 tbsp finely grated
   orange zest

**You will need a
12-hole cupcake tin**

Carrot and Cinnamon Cupcakes

These moist carrot cupcakes, spiced with a touch of cinnamon and nutmeg, are perfect for any occasion. I've always loved carrot cake and vegan versions are pretty easy to make because the carrots, as well as the rapeseed oil, keep them nice and moist.

Preheat the oven to 180°C fan, then either line the tin with cupcake cases or lightly grease the moulds with rapeseed oil.

In a large bowl, sift together the plain flour, baking powder, bicarbonate of soda, cinnamon, nutmeg and salt, then add the wholemeal flour. Add the carrots and sugar and set aside for 10 minutes to allow the carrots to moisten the flour.

In a separate bowl, mix together the rapeseed oil, milk and vanilla extract, then gently fold this into the dry ingredients, followed by the flax eggs and lemon juice.

Divide the batter between the cupcake cases or prepared moulds, so that they are half full, and bake in the oven for about 20 minutes or until a skewer inserted into the middle of one cupcake comes out clean. Remove from the oven and allow to cool in the tin for 5 minutes, then transfer the cakes to a wire rack to cool completely.

While the cupcakes are cooling, make the frosting. Place all the ingredients in a food mixer, using the smaller quantity of lemon juice, and blend until smooth and creamy. Alternatively, use an electric whisk to mix the ingredients together. If the frosting is too thick, add a little more lemon juice, bit by bit, until you reach the desired consistency. Spread the frosting on top of each of the cooled cupcakes and add a sprinkling of crushed walnuts to decorate. Store in a tin or other airtight container for up to 3 days.

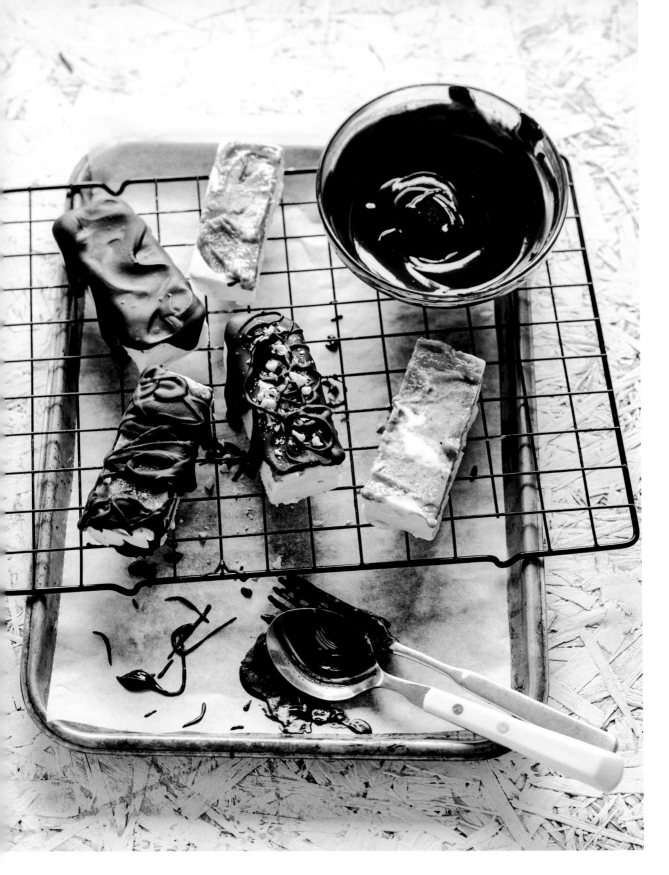

Puddings

Makes 6

1 × 350ml tub of vegan vanilla ice cream, softened
Handful of hazelnuts, crushed

For the date caramel sauce
6 pitted dates, roughly chopped
1 tsp vanilla extract
60ml vegan cream
Pinch of salt

For the chocolate coating
300g vegan dark chocolate, broken into squares
1 tbsp coconut oil
Pinch of salt

You will need
6 ice-cream moulds and 6 lolly sticks (optional) or a 13 × 23cm freezer-proof baking tray

Date Caramel Chocolate Ice Cream Bars

These bars are a summertime treat. Vegan ice cream is covered in a layer of salted date caramel sauce and then coated in chocolate. You can keep them as bars or add a lolly stick to make your own type of Magnum!

First make the date caramel sauce. If the dates are tough, soak them in warm water for 10 minutes, then drain. Add the dates to a high-speed blender or a food processor, along with the vanilla extract, cream and salt, and blend until smooth.

FOR THE NO-MOULD METHOD

Line the freezer-proof baking tray with baking paper, with enough excess overhanging the edges to allow you to lift the ice cream out of the tray once it has frozen. Spoon the ice cream into the prepared tray in a single layer about 2cm thick. You might need to let the ice cream melt slightly to create a smooth layer. Place in the freezer for 30 minutes to firm up, then add the date caramel sauce in a single layer and place back in the freezer for 2 hours to set.

Slice the sauce-coated ice cream into six rectangles and remove from the tray, then place, spaced apart, on a larger baking tray and return to the freezer to set for another hour. Follow the steps on the next page for coating the ice-cream bars in the chocolate mixture.

FOR THE ICE-CREAM MOULD METHOD

Spoon some ice cream into each of the ice-cream moulds, leaving a 5mm–1cm gap at the top of each mould for adding the date caramel sauce. You might need to let the ice cream melt slightly to create a smooth layer.

Continued on the next page

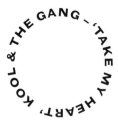

KOOL & THE GANG – 'TAKE MY HEART'

Insert a lolly stick (if using) into the centre of each mould and place in the freezer for 30 minutes to firm up.

Remove the moulds from the freezer, add some of the date caramel sauce to each mould and return to the freezer for 2 hours to set.

Fill a saucepan with water to a depth of 2–3cm and bring to a simmer, then reduce the heat to low. Place the chocolate in a heatproof bowl that will fit snugly on top of the pan without the water touching the base of the bowl. Stir the chocolate occasionally as it begins to soften, then remove the pan from the heat once the chocolate has melted and mix in the coconut oil and salt.

Gently remove the ice-cream bars from the moulds, lay on a freezer-proof baking tray lined with baking paper and place back in the freezer. When the ice-cream bars are completely frozen, remove one from the freezer and dip it into the melted chocolate, making sure the entire bar is covered – using a spoon to help if needed – and letting the excess chocolate drip off, then scatter with a little of the crushed hazelnuts. When all the bars have been coated, leave in the freezer until ready to serve.

Serves 9

200g pitted dates, chopped
    into small chunks
275ml plant-based milk
    (to make your own,
    see page 238)
200g self-raising flour
Pinch of salt
115g vegan butter, melted,
    plus extra for greasing

120ml maple syrup
1 tsp vanilla extract
1 tsp bicarbonate of soda
1 tbsp apple cider vinegar
Vegan vanilla ice cream,
    to serve

For the toffee sauce
200g soft dark brown sugar
150g vegan butter
100ml vegan cream
1 tsp vanilla extract

**You will need a
22cm square cake tin**

Sticky Toffee Pudding

The infamous, ever-so-British dessert! This deliciously moist pudding is incredible: the dates keep the cake nice and soft while also being a natural sweetener. Serve drizzled with an indulgent toffee sauce and with a scoop of vegan ice cream. And always serve warm for the ultimate sticky toffee pudding experience!

Preheat the oven to 180°C fan, then grease the cake tin with butter and line the base with baking paper.

Place the dates and milk in a saucepan set over a medium heat and cook for 7–10 minutes, stirring occasionally, until the dates soften, then remove from the heat.

Meanwhile, sift the flour and salt into a large bowl. In a separate bowl, mix together the butter, maple syrup and vanilla extract, then whisk until smooth.

Once the dates have softened, add the bicarbonate of soda and the apple cider vinegar. Gently mix this into the butter and maple syrup mixture, then add to the bowl with the flour and carefully fold in to combine.

Pour the batter into the prepared cake tin and bake in the oven for 40 minutes or until a skewer inserted into the middle of the cake comes out clean.

Meanwhile, add all the ingredients for the toffee sauce to a saucepan, set over a low heat, and stir frequently until smooth.

Remove the cake from the oven, leaving it in the tin, and pierce the top in several places with a skewer, then run some of the toffee sauce over to soak in. Cut the pudding into squares and serve with more of the toffee sauce poured over and a dollop of ice cream.

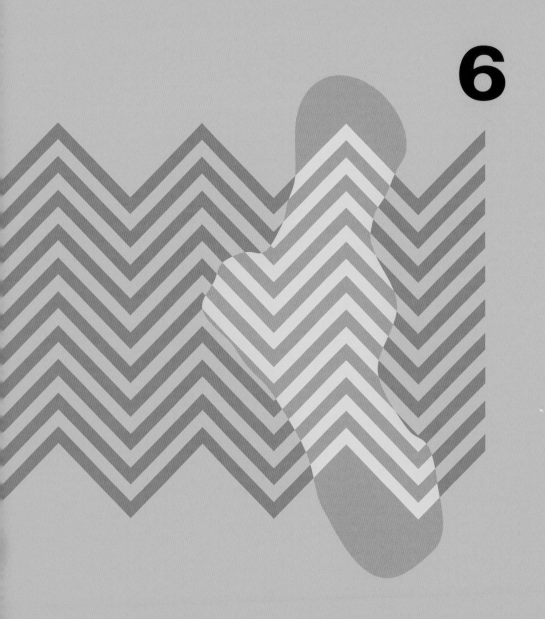

6

SMOOTHIES, JUICES AND HOT DRINKS

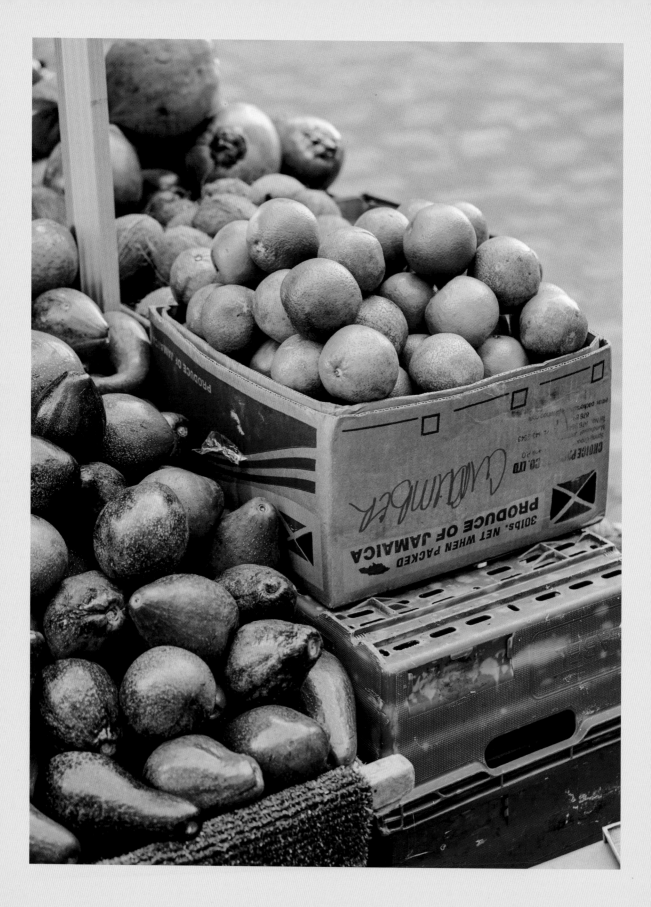

Smoothies, Juices and Hot Drinks

Smoothies are a go-to in the summer when I want a quick snack or a simple way to get some extra protein in me after a workout (using a protein powder) for some plant-based fuel. They're so simple and quick to blend together with a variety of different fruits. I like to keep fresh fruits in the freezer so I always have some fruit to work with.

There's also a fresh juice in this chapter, but don't worry if you don't have a juicer; you can mix fruits and vegetables in a high-speed blender and strain them – you can actually use the leftover pulp for making cakes as an egg replacement!

Serves 1

1–3 pitted dates (to taste)
1 banana, peeled
160g frozen mango
160g frozen pineapple
100g spinach
Thumb-sized piece of fresh
    root ginger, peeled and
    roughly chopped
240ml coconut water
1 tsp moringa powder
1 tbsp chia seeds

Tropical Moringa Smoothie

If the dates are hard, soak them in a bowl of warm water for 5–10 minutes before blending.

Place all the ingredients except the chia seeds in a high-speed blender or food processor and blitz until smooth. Pour into a large glass and mix in the chia seeds to serve.

Don't let the green colour fool you: this nutrient-rich tropical smoothie, sweetened with mango, pineapple and banana, is so delicious and refreshing! The coconut water maximises hydration while the chia seeds give a lovely smooth texture. One of my favourite ways to get in extra greens such as spinach, which can sometimes be a bit bitter, is to mix them in with tropical fruits. To make this even easier, try freezing the fresh ripe fruit ahead of time so that you always have some handy for making delicious smoothies and juices.

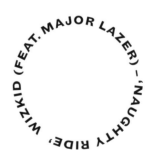

WIZKID (FEAT. MAJOR LAZER) – 'NAUGHTY RIDE',

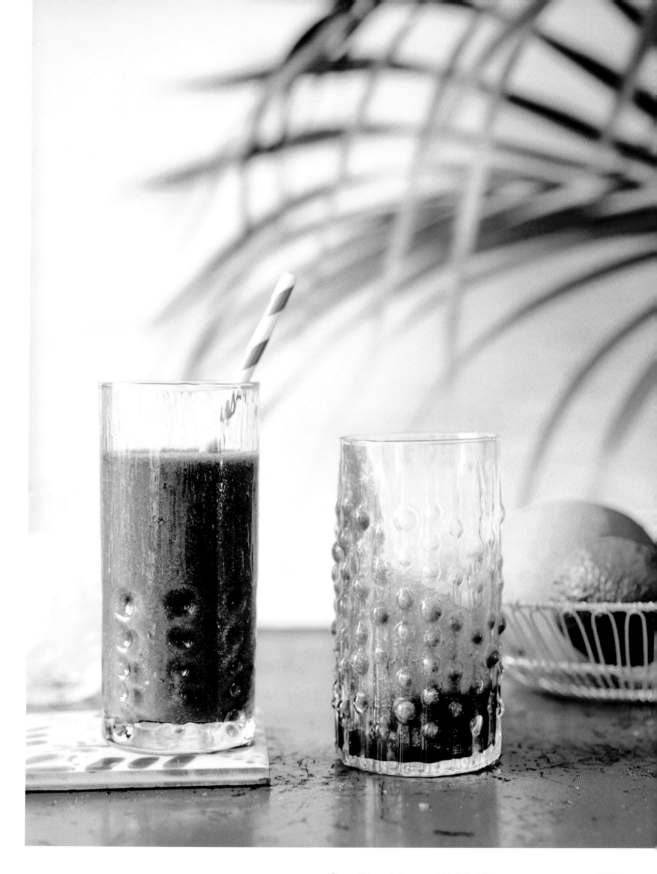

Smoothies, Juices and Hot Drinks

2–4 pitted dates (to taste)
40g rolled oats
150g frozen mixed berries
1 banana, peeled
150ml plant-based milk
(to make your own,
see page 238)
1 scoop of protein powder
(following packet
instructions for
dosage; optional)

1 raw beetroot, peeled
3 carrots
2 eating apples,
peeled and cored
Thumb-sized piece of fresh
root ginger, peeled
Juice of ½ lemon

Breakfast On-the-go Berry Shake

Do you struggle to find time to sit down and eat breakfast before leaving the house? This smoothie is a great way to fill you up on your way out the door. Simply mix everything together in a blender – and go! The oats and optional protein powder will give you that extra boost to start the day.

If the dates are hard, soak in a bowl of warm water for 5–10 minutes before blending.

Place all the ingredients in a high-speed blender or food processor and blitz until smooth. Pour into a glass and serve.

Beet and Carrot Juice

Juicing is a great way to get a variety of fruits and vegetables into your system, especially in the summer when you want a nice, cool refreshing drink that's full of natural nutrients. This ruby-red beetroot juice is super-simple to make: the carrots, apples and root ginger bring it alive with a refreshing sweetness and subtle spiciness. If you don't have a juicer, you can blend the ingredients instead and then push them through a fine-meshed sieve. You can reserve the pulp for adding to cakes or smoothies.

Wash all the ingredients and place in a juicer, then juice them according to the manufacturer's instructions. Pour into a glass, add the lemon juice and mix in with a spoon before drinking.

Serves 1

240ml oat milk (to make your own, see page 238)
1½ tbsp raw cacao powder
1–2 tbsp date syrup

1 tsp chaga mushroom powder (following packet instructions for dosage)
Pinch of salt

Chaga Mushroom Hot Chocolate

A delicious, warming hot chocolate with a twist! Said to have been used for centuries to boost stamina and the immune system, chaga mushroom is regarded by some as the king of medicinal mushrooms due to its powerful antioxidant properties. If you don't have date syrup you can use any sweetener of your choice, such as agave or maple syrup. And for an equally delicious regular hot chocolate, just leave out the mushroom powder.

Place all the ingredients in a saucepan, adding the smaller quantity of date syrup, and set over a medium heat. Heat until piping hot, using a whisk to break up any cocoa lumps and stirring until smooth. Taste for sweetness, adding the rest of the date syrup if needed.

Pour into a mug and serve warm.

7

BASICS ○ ○ ○
AND ⋀⋁⋀⋁
ESSENTIALS

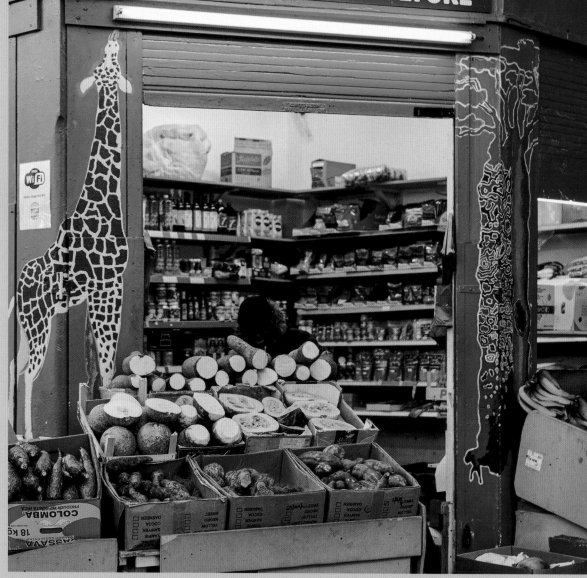

Basics and Essentials

This chapter includes a variety of recipes that I use every day as a basis for making meals, as well as things like nut butters, which I consider a store cupboard essential as I love them.

You'll find a nice long list of options for replacing eggs in different recipes, whether you want fluffier bakes and cakes or soft and moist ones.

I use plant-based milks for my granola or porridge and in tea and coffee. There are so many different options that you can make using nuts, seeds or even oats, so I like to mix it up. You can also turn them into delicious chocolate milks or berry milks. Cashew nuts are my favourite for a really creamy consistency – so good for hot chocolate!

I've also included some really simple nut butter recipes. When I want a pretty immediate snack I always turn to nut butters: I spread them on toast or crackers, add them to smoothies, or dip dates into them – so good! They're really handy: make a big jar and munch on it over the week.

Egg Replacements

Eggs are quite a key ingredient in non-vegan baking but there are easy ways to replace them in a vegan diet. Below are a few different replacements for your cakes, bakes and general recipes. Some are best for binding ingredients together, some are best for adding moisture and some add fluffiness, which is good for cakes, pancakes and things of that nature.

Each recipe makes the equivalent of 1 egg

FLAX EGG
Best for binding.

1 tbsp ground flaxseeds
3 tbsp water

Mix together the ground flaxseeds and water in a bowl and allow to sit for at least 10 minutes until it becomes gel-like in consistency.

CHICKPEA EGG
Best for binding.

3 tbsp chickpea flour
3 tbsp water

In a bowl, mix together the chickpea flour and water until smooth.

BAKING SODA EGG
For fluffier baked goods.

1 tsp bicarbonate of soda
1 tbsp fresh lemon juice

In a bowl, mix the bicarbonate of soda with the lemon juice until smooth.

BANANA EGG

Best for adding moisture.

½ banana

Use a fork to mash the banana into a purée.

FRUIT PURÉE EGG

Best for adding moisture.

3 tbsp shop-bought apple,
    pumpkin or sweet potato purée

Simply add to a dish as specified in the
particular recipe.

CHIA EGG

Best for binding.

1 tbsp chia seeds
3 tbsp water

Mix the chia seeds and water in a bowl and set aside for
10 minutes or so until it becomes gel-like in consistency.

AQUAFABA

A replacement for egg whites, such as in meringues
(see page 203) or mayonnaise (see page 189).

3 tbsp aquafaba (liquid from a tin
    of chickpeas), whipped

To use as a binder, lightly whip until foamy. For use in
mayonnaise or meringues, whip into stiff peaks (peaks
that hold their shape when you lift the whisk out of the
bowl), taking care not to over-whip.

Plant-based Milks

Making your own plant-based milks is a great way to cut down on waste, and use quality ingredients. Experiment with a variety of different nuts and plants; you can adjust the sweetness and how creamy you want it to be for that perfect cup of tea, cereal, smoothie, hot chocolate or whatever you like to use plant-based milks for!

Once each milk has been blended, strain it through a muslin cloth into a bowl. Squeeze the cloth to extract all the liquid and discard the pulp left behind. Pour the milk into an airtight container and store in the fridge for up to 4 days.

ALMOND MILK

Makes about 1.5 litres
200g whole raw almonds
1 litre water

Cover the almonds in water in a bowl and leave to soak overnight or for a minimum of 10–12 hours.

Drain the almonds, then tip them into a high-speed blender or a food processor, add the water and blitz until smooth before straining into a bowl (see introduction).

OAT MILK

Makes about 1.25 litres
100g rolled oats
1 litre water
Pinch of salt

Cover the oats in water in a bowl and leave to soak for at least 1 hour.

Drain the oats, then tip them into a high-speed blender or a food processor, add the water and the salt and blitz until smooth. Take care to not over-mix as the heat from the blender/processor blades can cause the oats to warm up and begin to cook, thus changing the texture of the milk and making it slimy. Once blended, strain the milk into a bowl (see introduction).

CASHEW NUT MILK

Makes about 1 litre
150g raw cashew nuts
720ml water
Pinch of pink Himalayan salt (optional)

Cover the cashews in water in a bowl and leave to soak for 2 hours.

Drain the cashews, then tip them into a high-speed blender or a food processor, add the water and the salt (if using) and blitz until smooth before straining into a bowl (see introduction).

CHOCOLATE MILK

Makes 750ml–1 litre
1–3 pitted dates (to taste)
750ml–1 litre Plant-based Milk (see opposite)
2–3 tbsp raw cacao powder (to taste)
Pinch of salt

If the dates are tough, first soak them in warm water for 5 minutes, then drain. Place the dates in a high-speed blender or food processor, along with the remaining ingredients, and blitz until smooth, then store in an airtight container in the fridge for up to 4 days.

BERRY MILK

Makes about 1 litre
750ml–1 litre Plant-based Milk (see opposite)
140g fresh berries (such as raspberries, strawberries or blueberries)
2–3 tbsp maple syrup (to taste)

Place all the ingredients in a high-speed blender or food processor and whizz until smooth, then store in an airtight container in the fridge for up to 4 days.

Nut and Seed Butters

Nut butters are great to have in your cupboard for when you want a quick snack. Nut butter on toast is one of my main go-tos when I'm peckish and want something hassle-free. You can also add nut butters to smoothies or even use them as dips for dates or bananas – so delicious. You will need a strong food processor for the nuts and seeds to break them down well, but the butters are easy to make! And if you make your own you can control what goes into them and add additional sweetness or more oil for a looser consistency. I've included a sunflower seed butter recipe for those of you who have nut allergies. Sunflower seeds have less oil than most nuts which means you need to add a little; this creates a really tasty, rich butter which you can use as an alternative to nut butters.

ALMOND/PEANUT BUTTER

Makes 400g

400g raw almonds or unsalted peanuts
2–3 tbsp coconut oil or other
   neutral-flavoured oil (optional)
Pink Himalayan salt or sea salt
1–2 tbsp maple syrup (optional)

Preheat the oven to 180°C fan. Spread the nuts out on a baking sheet in a single layer and roast for 10–15 minutes, until lightly browned, then remove from the oven, tip them into a bowl and allow them to cool completely.

Once cool, place the nuts in a food processor and blitz. First they will break down, then slowly the oils will start to be released, turning the mix into a smooth, creamy almond or peanut butter. For a smoother, more loose consistency, add 1 tablespoon of coconut oil at a time until you reach your desired consistency. Season with salt to taste. For additional sweetness, add maple syrup to taste, and blitz until combined. Place in a sterilised jar (see page 175) and store for up to a week.

SUNFLOWER SEED BUTTER

Makes 400g

400g sunflower seeds
3–4 tbsp coconut oil
Pink Himalayan salt or sea salt
2 tbsp maple syrup (optional)

Preheat the oven to 180°C fan. Spread the seeds out on a baking sheet in a single layer – you may need to use two sheets – and roast for 10 minutes until they are lightly browned.

Allow the seeds to cool completely then place in a food processor and blitz. Sunflower seeds can take a little longer to process than nuts, so blending can take up to 10 minutes. The seeds will break down into clumps, then a sand-like consistency. Once the seeds have broken down – after about 5 minutes – start to add 3 tablespoons of the coconut oil while the food processor is still blitzing. Add more coconut oil if the seed butter is still too thick. Season with a hint of salt and if you want to, add the maple syrup for a little sweetness. Place in a sterilised jar (see page 175) and store for up to a week.

Makes about 335g

250g whole hazelnuts
60g icing sugar
Pinch of salt
200g vegan dark chocolate,
    at least 70% cocoa solids
1 tbsp coconut oil

Chocolate Hazelnut Spread

Hazelnuts and chocolate are probably one of the best combos! This simple, incredibly addictive recipe makes a delicious, rich chocolate hazelnut spread, like a slightly healthier version of Nutella. Spread this across a slice of toasted bread, or add it to smoothies! You can use store-bought, ready-roasted hazelnuts for ease if you don't want to roast them yourself. Once made, make sure you keep it in an airtight jar and store it at room temperature. The spread does thicken over time, especially if you live in cold climates where room temperature is pretty cold, but it's still smooth enough to spread across bread. If you choose to store it in the fridge, it will keep slightly longer but will also solidify and will need to be warmed slightly to get that smooth spread.

Preheat the oven to 180°C fan. Spread the hazelnuts on a baking tray and roast in the oven for 5–10 minutes, tossing them halfway through and checking regularly to ensure that they don't burn. Remove from the oven, place on a clean tea towel and gently rub to remove the skins.

Place the skinned hazelnuts in a high-speed blender or food processor and blitz until the nuts turn into a very smooth oily butter.

While blending, add the sugar and salt and blend until all the ingredients have been incorporated and the mixture is smooth. Turn off the machine and taste for seasoning, adding more salt if needed, then transfer.

Fill a saucepan with water to a depth of 2–3cm and bring to a simmer, then reduce the heat to low. Place the chocolate in a heatproof bowl that fits snugly on top of the pan without the water touching the base. Stir the chocolate occasionally as it begins to soften, then remove the pan from the heat once the chocolate has melted and mix in the coconut oil, then remove the bowl from the pan.

Pour the hazelnut mixture into the chocolate, stirring slowly to combine. Pour the spread into a sterilised jar (see page 175), seal with a lid and chill in the fridge before using. Store at room temperature for up to 5 days.

Store Cupboard Glossary

Here I've given you a short guide to lots of the ingredients that appear in the recipes, some things you may already be familiar with and are simply ingredients I use a lot in vegan cooking; some you may not have come across, such as a few of the Caribbean seasonings. Some of the powders I use to add to my food are listed separately because these are totally optional extras, for you to choose whether you want to make them part of your diet or not.

ACKEE, TINNED

Ackee is a fruit native to West Africa. It was introduced to Jamaica in the 1770s and Jamaica is now home to the famous ackee and saltfish dish. It is subtle in taste but absorbs flavour really well. Unripe and unprepared ackee can be poisonous, so it is sold tinned under strict guidelines for safe eating. My go-to brand is Dunn's River Ackee; I buy their tinned ackee in water, which you can find in large supermarkets like Sainsbury's and Tesco as well as small independent food stores.

ALFALFA SPROUTS

Alfalfa sprouts come from the shoots of the alfalfa plant harvested before they grow into the full plant. Despite their small size, they're rich in antioxidants, vitamins and minerals. I love adding them to salads and sandwiches – they're slightly crunchy with a mild nutty taste.

AQUAFABA

The cooking liquid from chickpeas and other legumes; I like to use chickpea liquid. The easiest way to get hold of it is to pop open a can of chickpeas and the liquid there is your aquafaba. Its composition gives it amazing emulsifying, foaming and binding abilities. You can whip it up like egg whites and make silky mayo, meringues and light baked goods. I love to whip up a quick vegan mayonnaise (see page 189), especially when I use a can of chickpeas to make my chickpea Chuna (see page 150) – it's really simple, with such minimal ingredients, and tastes so good.

CACAO POWDER, RAW

Although cacao powder and cocoa powder both come from the same raw cacao bean they're very different. Cocoa powder, which you'll see a lot of around the supermarkets and in chocolate bars, is made differently to raw cacao powder. It's processed at high temperatures which removes a lot of the natural nutrients and often has sugars and other ingredients added to it. Whether I make a hot chocolate or just want a chocolatey porridge, I like to stick to raw cacao powder to get my chocolate fix because the lower temperatures at which it's processed mean it retains the cacao bean's nutrients. I always recommend buying Fairtrade and organic raw cacao.

CHIA SEEDS

Chia seeds are little edible seeds from the desert plant *Salvia hispanica*. They're a great source of omega-3 fatty acids, proteins, fibre, antioxidants and more. The word is that ancient Aztecs and Mayans used chia seeds as their sources of energy. Chia seeds are a personal favourite of mine. I always pop them in my porridge and I love making a fresh smoothie then adding chia seeds right at the end; they absorb some of the liquid and turn silky, adding texture and thickening the smoothie.

CHICKPEA FLOUR

Chickpea flour, also known as gram flour, is made by grinding dried chickpeas. It is rich in protein and fibre and is a great gluten-free alternative to plain flour with a mild earthy and nutty flavour. You can find it in most health food stores and large supermarkets. I sometimes use it as an egg replacement to help bind ingredients together, or I just use it to make things like waffles or Caribbean fried bakes.

COCONUT AMINOS
(REPLACEMENT FOR SOY SAUCE)

Coconut aminos is a salty-savoury sauce made from fermented coconut sap. It is a great replacement for soy sauce if you don't eat soy or gluten, as although it is not as rich as dark soy sauce it has a similar flavour to light soy sauce and surprisingly doesn't taste like coconut.

GARLIC GRANULES

Garlic granules are dehydrated minced garlic and are a quick and easy way to add garlic flavour to your meals.

HARISSA / ROSE HARISSA PASTE

Harissa is a spicy paste that originates in North Africa. Recipes vary across different regions and the Middle East, but essentially it is a deliciously layered chilli sauce made with roasted red peppers, hot chilli peppers, lemon, garlic, spices and herbs, from coriander seeds to rose and saffron. You can purchase it in most large supermarkets and add it to couscous or pasta, dip fresh bread into it or spread it across grid-dled or roast vegetables for a tasty aromatic chilli kick.

HEARTS OF PALM

Hearts of palm are a vegetable harvested from the centre of certain palm trees. The flavour is very savoury, similar to artichoke but far more subtle and delicate.

I love using them in recipes which traditionally call for fish, such as fish cakes or ackee and saltfish. You can buy them tinned in most large supermarkets or they're easy to find online.

HEMP SEEDS

Hemp seeds are packed with protein and essential fatty acids, including omega-3 and omega-6, and are rich in antioxidants. They're slightly nutty and creamy in taste. I normally sprinkle them on to salads and breakfast meals like toasts and porridge for some extra nutrients.

JACKFRUIT, TINNED

Jackfruit is native to southwest India. You can get tinned jackfruit from most large supermarkets nowadays or Asian supermarkets. Jackfruit has a subtle salty and savoury taste and when pulled apart it is stringy – like pulled meat or flaked fish. It's a great texture to play around with when cooking vegan meals as it can absorb flavours really well. I love using it to make fish-like recipes.

LIQUID SMOKE
(CAN BE REPLACED WITH SOY SAUCE /TAMARI SAUCE / COCONUT AMINOS)

In general liquid smoke is made by concentrating the flavour of wood smoke. Different brands may add additional flavours. As it stands today Stubb's Hickory Liquid Smoke and Colgin Natural Hickory Liquid Smoke are listed as vegan-friendly and are ones I turn to. They add a smoky flavour to meals, which I love, especially in the summer when grilling mushrooms and aubergines.

NORI FLAKES / SHEETS

Nori sheets are made by shredding edible seaweed and pressing them into thin sheets. You can buy them toasted or plain and they add really tasty sea-like flavours to meals. I use them a lot for creating vegan versions of dishes that were originally made from seafood, like saltfish or smoked salmon (see pages 74 and 59).

NUTRITIONAL YEAST
Nutritional yeast is a type of deactivated yeast usually found as flakes or in powdered form in most natural health food shops and some larger supermarkets as well as online. It has a mild nutty and savoury cheese-like flavour. Nutritional yeast is great to use as a replacement for Parmesan when sprinkled on pasta or added to creamy sauces to give them extra depth of flavour.

ONION POWDER
Onion powder is dehydrated ground onion. It's great for seasoning when you've run out of onions or want to add quick and easy flavour to sauces and foods.

QUINOA FLOUR
Quinoa flour is made by grinding quinoa seeds into a fine consistency. It's a great way to add extra essential proteins and amino acids to meals; you can even use it like a protein powder in smoothies. I like to make pancakes and waffles with quinoa flour as they're filling, nutritious but still light and delicious.

SCOTCH BONNET CHILLI PEPPERS
Scotch bonnet chilli peppers are fiery with a distinct taste that has a hint of sweetness alongside the spice. I've grown more addicted to them over time. They're found in many Caribbean and West African recipes but if you can't get hold of them, you can use regular red chillies to your preferred level of spiciness. They're hot, so if you are new to them, start with a little, maybe a quarter of the pepper for a curry dish.

TAHINI
Tahini is a paste made from sesame seeds which is widely used in Middle Eastern cuisines. It is creamy and mildly nutty. It's great for baking and making dressings. You can buy light or dark varieties but my personal preference is light tahini. There is a big difference between good and bad tahini: bad tahini can be quite bitter. You want to find one that is rich, smooth and loose. I've tried quite a few brands and would recommend AL Taj tahini or authentic ones from independent sellers. Interestingly, one of my favourite tahinis comes all the way from Japan. While my mum was there a friend recommended it to her and it was so good! Unfortunately I can't remember the name of it – I'll need to go to Japan myself one day.

TAMARI SAUCE
Tamari is a Japanese version of soy sauce. It can be a bit darker in colour and richer with a less salty taste than soy sauce and is a great gluten-free alternative.

TAMARIND PASTE
Tamarind paste is made from the pulp inside the pods of the tamarind fruit tree. It's used a lot in Thai cooking as well as Indian and Mexican cuisines. It's a little sticky in texture and sour in taste so it's good to balance it with something sweet, which is why I love it in a good pad Thai recipe. You can buy fresh tamarind pulp which can be richer in flavour but can be hard to find in your everyday supermarket, in which case tamarind paste works well.

VANILLA BEAN PASTE
Vanilla bean paste is made by blending vanilla extract with vanilla beans and seeds. It is great to use as a quick substitute for fresh vanilla pods. It adds a rich flavour to cakes, cookies, ice creams and more. It's always worth checking the ingredients to make sure you're buying pure vanilla bean paste as some are blended with fillers.

VEGAN DARK CHOCOLATE

Dark chocolate should in theory be vegan but a lot aren't necessarily so keep an eye on the ingredients list for added dairy just to be sure. (As it sounds, milk chocolate does have dairy added.)

VEGAN MINCE

There are different types of vegan mince available. Some are made from textured soy protein or wheat gluten and some are made using a combination of grains, such as quinoa, buckwheat and so on. I always try and look out for ones with minimal ingredients and flavourings and let the vegan mince absorb the flavours I cook it in. A few brands to note are Vivera, Clearspring, Fry's, Waitrose and Tesco, with more coming into play every day!

VEGAN BUTTER

There are quite a few spreads out there to replace butters – they are simply made from plant-based oils, such as sunflower oil, avocado oil and so on. I like using Flora's dairy-free spread which is vegan – the taste and texture are how I remember butter and I love it. I find it good for baking too.

VEGAN ALTERNATIVES TO YOGHURT

When it comes to yoghurts my favourites are made from coconut, though you can also find oat, almond, cashew and soy yoghurts.

POWDERS

AÇAI POWDER

Açai powder comes from açai berries, which are native to Brazil and northern South America. Deep purple in colour the berries are packed with antioxidants and are super-nutritious. If you can get fresh açai berries I highly recommend adding them to smoothies. I've found it hard getting fresh açai berries in the UK that don't have added sugars so I opt for an organic powdered form.

CHAGA MUSHROOM POWDER

Made from chaga mushrooms grown on birch trees around North America, Eastern Europe and Asia. The powerful mushroom is super rich in antioxidants. I love adding a little to smoothies and hot chocolate for some extra nutrients.

MORINGA POWDER

Moringa powder comes from the leaves of the *Moringa oleifera* tree, which is native to North India. It has been praised for its health benefits for thousands of years. It's rich in antioxidants and has lots of vitamins and minerals. I like adding moringa to pancakes, waffles and smoothies. As you use it in such small quantities it doesn't really add a taste to food, just the nutrients.

PROTEIN POWDER

An option for anyone wanting to include some more protein in their diet. There are lots of different high-quality sources of plant-based protein that you can get in powdered form, such as rice, hemp, soy, pea, chia and many more. You can add them straight to smoothies and pancake batters, or the unflavoured varieties can also be used to thicken soups and stews for a quick and easy protein top-up. Opt for pure natural powders with minimal added ingredients and ideally organic.

Conversion Chart

All my recipes have been tested in metric measurements and I use a fan oven. If your oven is not fan-assisted, you may have to increase the cooking time or temperature by about 10 per cent.

Here are some conversions for those who like to use imperial measurements (i.e. ounces and pints) or American cup measurements. Please do bear in mind that converting from weight to volume (i.e. cups) is not an exact science, so if in doubt, use the weight!

WEIGHT

Metric	Imperial
10g	½oz
25g	1oz
50g	2oz
75g	3oz
110g	4oz
150g	5oz
175g	6oz
200g	7oz
225g	8oz
250g	9oz
275g	10oz
350g	12oz
450g	1lb
700g	1lb 8oz
900g	2lb

VOLUME

Imperial	Metric
2fl oz	55ml
3fl oz	75ml
5fl oz (¼ pint)	150ml
10fl oz (½ pint)	275ml
1 pint	570ml
1¼ pints	725ml
1¾ pints	1 litre
2 pints	1.2 litres
2½ pints	1.5 litres
4 pints	2.25 litres

OVEN TEMPERATURES

Gas Mark	°F	°C
1	275°F	140°C
2	300°F	150°C
3	325°F	170°C
4	350°F	180°C
5	375°F	190°C
6	400°F	200°C
7	425°F	220°C
8	450°F	230°C
9	475°F	240°C

AMERICAN CUP CONVERSIONS

American	Imperial	Metric
1 cup flour	5oz	150g
1 cup caster/granulated sugar	8oz	225g
1 cup brown sugar	6oz	175g
1 cup vegan butter	8oz	225g
1 cup sultanas/raisins	7oz	200g
1 cup ground almonds	4oz	110g
1 cup golden syrup	12oz	350g
1 cup uncooked rice	7oz	200g

LIQUID CONVERSIONS

Imperial	Metric	American
½fl oz	15ml	1 tbsp
1fl oz	30ml	⅛ cup
2fl oz	60ml	¼ cup
4fl oz	120ml	½ cup
8fl oz	240ml	1 cup
16fl oz	480ml	1 pint

Index

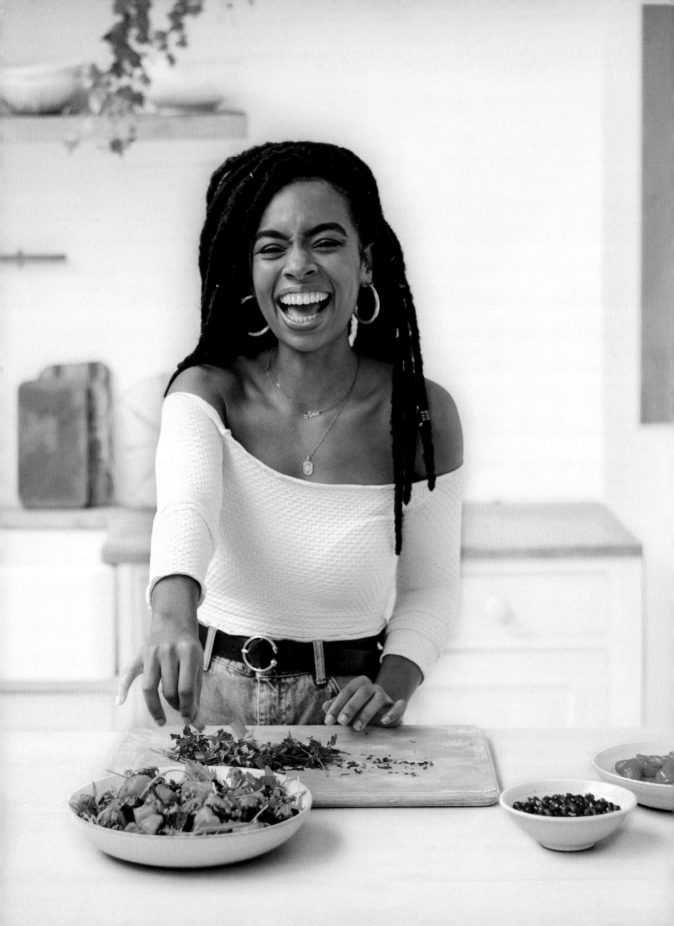

Acknowledgements

When I started my YouTube channel in 2017 I had no clue I'd be here in 2018 writing a cookbook. I don't quite know how to write my gratitude to all the amazing humans who have supported me, but here goes.

Firstly I'd like to thank my mum: you have always supported and encouraged every creative idea I've had. That belief in me has been monumental to getting here today and writing my first cookbook. I can't thank you enough for being my superhero, my idol and my strength, for showing me the capacity for hard work and always believing in my dreams!

Shout out to my big brother Remi, whom I've always looked up to. Seeing first-hand how you share your creativity with the world has always inspired me to try and share a little of mine. You're my role model and you probably don't even know it! Thank you for being my big brother, Buffy would be proud.

Thank you Gu (mam-gu, which means grandma in Welsh) for your huge heart that I am lucky enough to be part of and for telling everyone in the local supermarkets, cinemas, cafés and restaurants to check out my YouTube channel.

I would also like to thank my fairy godmother Alice; I knew from the first email and then meeting you that I was in safe, strong and inspiring hands, and my hype man Nora at Found – all this wouldn't be possible without you guys and the wonderful team. Thank you for believing in me!

To my Grandma Pat who cooked the best Sunday dinners for us and also shared her incredible cooking in schools, nursing homes and hospitals. Although I didn't know it at the time I know that my taste buds and love for cooking come from you.

To the amazing team at Ebury Press, thank you so much for being my publishers and giving me the opportunity to create a book that I can really call my own: from the recipes, to adding the music, to using my fabric prints – everything. I can't say thank you enough! It's been a real privilege to work with such an incredible team.

Liz and Max (Coco too): I had so much fun shooting the book with you; thank you for helping my vision come to life with your incredible talent and, of course, amazing company on those cold winter days.

A huge thank you to everyone who has been rocking with me on this journey, my YouTubers, my Instagrammers, my family, new friends and old friends; my heart is so full, thank you all!

In memory of my Grandma Pat.

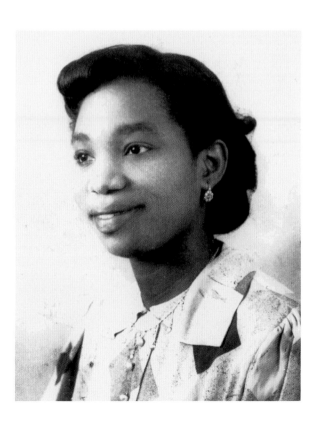

10 9 8 7 6 5 4 3 2 1

Published in 2019 by Ebury Press an imprint of Ebury Publishing,
20 Vauxhall Bridge Road, London SW1V 2SA

Ebury Press is part of the Penguin Random House group of companies
whose addresses can be found at global.penguinrandomhouse.com

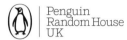

www.penguin.co.uk

A CIP catalogue record for this book is available from the British Library

ISBN 9781529104578

Design: Imagist
Photography: Haarala Hamilton
Food Styling: Frankie Unsworth
Food Stylist's Assistant: Izy Hossack
Prop Styling: Rebecca Newport

Colour origination by Altaimage Ltd, London
Printed and bound in Italy by LEGO S.p.A

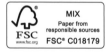

MIX
Paper from
responsible sources
FSC
www.fsc.org   FSC® C018179

Penguin Random House is committed to a sustainable future for our
business, our readers and our planet. This book is made from Forest
Stewardship Council® certified paper.

The information in this book has been compiled by way of general guidance
in relation to the specific subjects addressed, but it is not a substitute and not
to be relied on for medical, healthcare, pharmaceutical or other professional
advice on specific circumstances and in specific locations. Please consult
your GP before changing, stopping or starting any medical treatment. So far
as the author is aware the information given is correct and up to date as at
March 2019. Practice, laws and regulations all change, and the reader should
obtain up to date professional advice on any such issue. The author and the
publishers disclaim, as far as the law allows, any liability arising directly or
indirectly from the use or misuse of the information contained in this book.

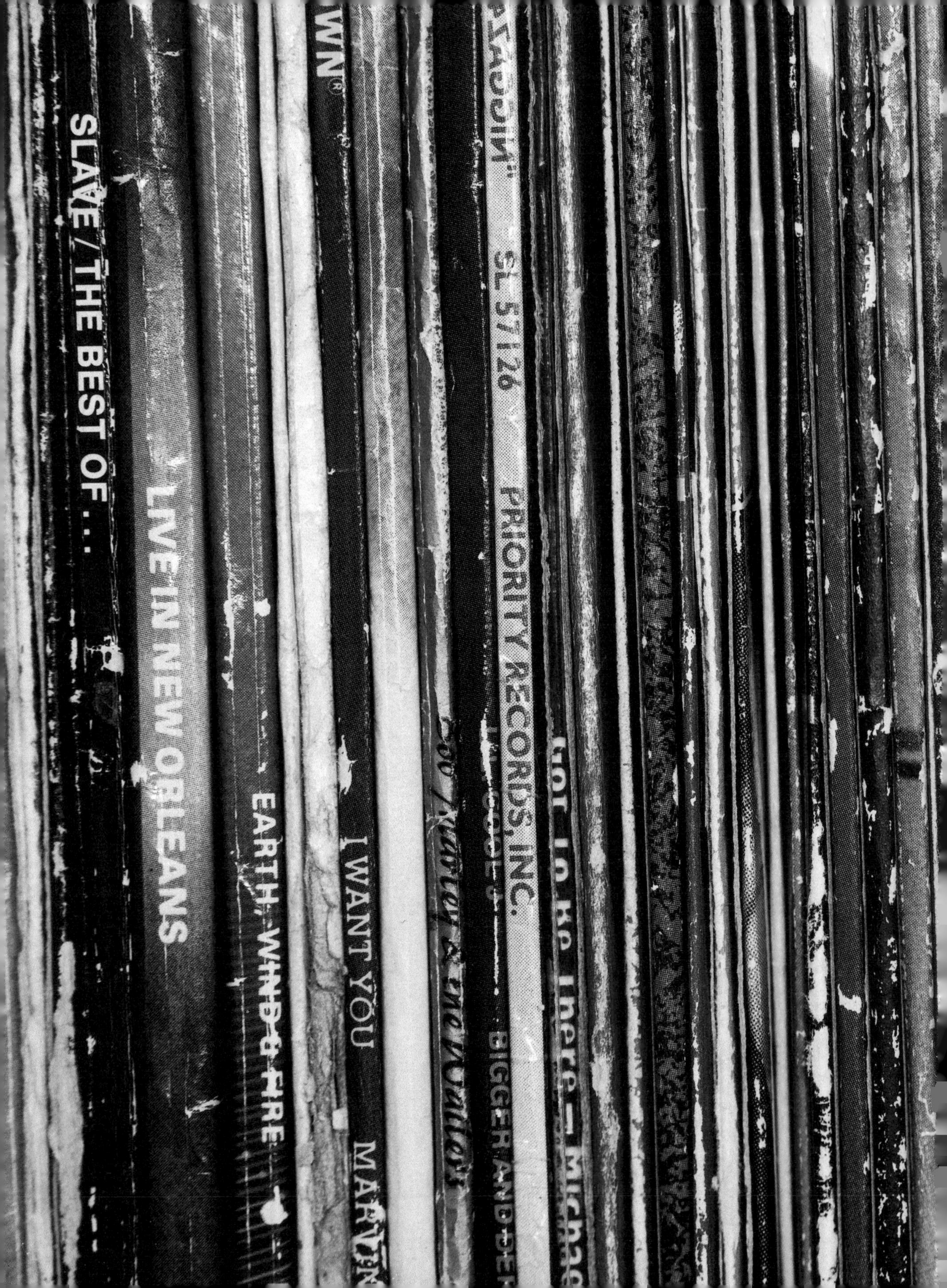

SLAVE / THE BEST OF ...

LIVE IN NEW ORLEANS

EARTH, WIND & FIRE

I WANT YOU

MARVIN

WN

ALADDIN

SL 57126

PRIORITY RECORDS, INC.

Bob Marley & the Wailers

Got To Be There — Michael

BIGGER AND DEF